A Diet Book For Weight Loss Success

James Atkinson

JIMSHEALTHANDMUSCLE.COM

BY: JBA Publishing
http://www.JimsHealthAndMuscle.com
jim@jimshealthandmuscle.com

A Diet Book for Weight Loss Success
Copyright © 2021 by James Atkinson
All Rights Reserved.

No part of this book may be reproduced or transmitted in any form or by any means, electronic, mechanical, photocopying, recording, or otherwise, without prior written permission of James Atkinson, except for brief quotations in critical reviews or articles.

Requests for permission to make copies of any part of this book should be submitted to James Atkinson at jim@jimshealthandmuscle.com

DISCLAIMER

Although the author and publisher have made every effort to ensure that the information contained in this book was accurate at the time of release, the author and publisher do not assume and hereby disclaim any liability to any party for any loss, damage, or disruption caused by errors or omissions in this book, whether such errors or omissions result from negligence, accident, or any other cause.

First published in 2021 / First printed in 2021 / First edition 2021

Copyright © 2021 JimsHealthAndMuscle.com

All rights reserved.

CONTENTS

"Why the diet book Jim?" 1

No diet beats education 2

Taking it to the extreme… 7

"Weight loss" or "Fat loss?" Mind-Set Revelations. 14

4 proven steps for successful diet creation TLDR 18

What's the best diet? It's a learning process 22

The calorie deficit vs other diet ideas. 27

Level 1 - Four steps to weight loss & diet success 31

Of which food labels? 42

Meal prep and "one pot cooking" 46

How much of a snack is this? 53

Water & your body, an easy tweak for maximum return 58

Exercise & diet for weight loss 64

Your very own companion guide 67

A nod to body types & genetics 69

SECTION 2 – Creating Your Diet 75

Introduction to section 2 76

Step 1 - Start your food diary 78

Step 2 - Set your goals 90

Step 3 - Plan your meals & water 95

Step 4 - Plan your exercise 98

Level 2 (Advanced planning and macros) 102

Keep going! Optimise for success. 112

Thank you and goodnight! 113

Motivation is the driving force! 115

"Why the diet book Jim?"

"There are many diet theories that will give the same results and there is so much confusion on weight loss diets. So I wanted to write a guide that focuses on the "basics done well". Everything in this diet book will apply to most, if not all. I hope that it gives you a base to work from, shows you that basic knowledge, a willingness to learn and a little upfront work can lead to truly amazing results.

Above all, I hope this book leaves you with a feeling of empowerment and positivity to set you up for exponential success with weight loss."

No diet beats education

When someone new to weight loss comes to me and asks me to write them a diet plan, my motivation to help always sparks! This is the breakthrough and shift in mind-set that they need, and this decision to make positive changes to lifestyle is where every success story starts, bar none!

This was the first step that the guy who has been overweight for his entire life took before becoming a fitness model. This was the first step that the self-proclaimed "Fat funny girl" took on her journey to becoming a competing figure contestant. This was the step that the guy who suffered with type 2 diabetes took before using diet and exercise to reduce his body fat by 60%, and this is the step that most of us will take at least once during our lifetimes.

I love the start of a success story and always jump at the opportunity to help because I know what we can achieve through correct diet and exercise. Unbelievable and impressive body transformations are not the only potential because the journey of achieving positive physical success has several side effects.

Arguably, the side effect that has the most impact on a success story is not the physical progress, but it is in the building of strength of character that is woven into the personal experience of the entire process.

This is really powerful stuff. I know because fitness success has built the character that I have today. If I'd not achieved what I have in fitness, I would not have had the confidence to quit the job I hated to set a business up for myself, I would not have had the conviction to stick to my goals when things got tough and I most definitely would not be writing this now, or have written any book, be it fitness related or otherwise.

When you actually hit a fitness or diet goal, you achieve far more than physical results, your horizon becomes broader in every direction; you believe in yourself a lot more; you believe that you can achieve all sorts of things that you never would have dreamed possible before, and now, you go after your dreams with conviction, as you know that anything is possible.

This is one reason that I get so motivated when someone comes to me for help with diet or exercise, I want everyone to experience this for themselves; I don't just want to give someone a list of food to eat; I want to empower people to change their lives and pass all of my knowledge and experience over so they can soak it up and get to the success as soon as possible.

If I just gave everyone who asked me for a diet plan a list of food to eat, I know that nine times out of 10, this would not be followed and would be a massive waste of time for all involved and even for the one person who followed this, they would not get a lot of value from it. This is not me guessing, this is from my actual life experience and it is in fact one of the last things that we should do.

If you were to follow a well-designed weight-loss diet plan to the letter, you would get results, and this is a win, but this path is a narrow one. I say it's narrow because as soon as you are in a position where you can't get some of the food on your list or you decide you don't like something on the list anymore, things can easily, and very quickly fall apart.

I've said many times before that the fitness, weight loss, diet journey or whatever you want to call it is not a straight path that's clear of obstacles so if you can equip yourself with the right tools for this journey from the outset, the twists, turns and obstacles will not throw you off or trip you up.

The most useful tool is by far Knowledge and education on nutrition when it comes to long term sustainable diet and body composition change.

Basic knowledge about food and nutrition is all that you need to create sustainable, long-term eating habits that really make a difference in weight management, body composition and ultimately a healthier, happier life.

This book is a practical guide, and it has all the information that you need to succeed with diet and weight loss. There are however practical steps, planning and tracking that need to be undertaken if you are to get the most from your efforts.

I have created a companion guide that runs directly alongside this book for you to make all the necessary planning, prep and tracking your own in the form of a physical notebook and journal.

"A diet book for weight loss success: The workbook and Journal "is the perfect daily, weekly and monthly companion to take on your weight loss transformation journey. The companion guide has all the necessary tracking charts, lists, motivational help and lots of extras inside to help you stay motivated, organised and keep you on track for fitness success!

If you would like to take advantage of this valuable resource, you can grab it:

HERE if you are in the US

HERE if you are in the UK

Or you can type this into the search bar on Amazon:

"A diet book for weight loss success: The workbook"

If you want to have your plan written down, organised, and ready to go by the time you've finished reading this book, empower yourself with the companion guide!

A DIET BOOK
FOR WEIGHT LOSS
SUCCESS

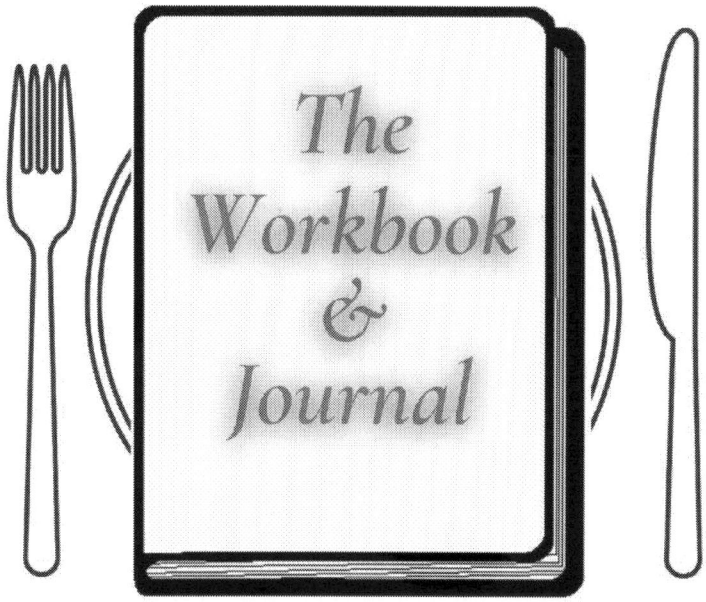
The Workbook & Journal

JAMES ATKINSON

So grab the companion guide to set yourself up for even more success from the start, and while you wait for the delivery, you can get started with this guide in preparation.

Taking it to the extreme...

> *"The effort you put in is relative to the result you get.*
>
> *If you want more, put more effort in"*

5:45 am and the familiar sound of the morning alarm brings me out of a deep sleep, just like it did yesterday morning and the day before that. It feels like this has been the way of things for as far back as I can remember. In fact, it's only been about twelve weeks, but as I can now see, twelve weeks will make a big difference in health and fitness if you really throw yourself at a goal and stay committed.

I get out of bed and head over to my workout clothes that I prepared the night before and get dressed before heading to the kitchen to drink a pint of water. It's then a trip out in the world for a 45 minute fat burning cardio session.

There are two things that I can guarantee after a cardio session like this; One – I will sweat and will need a shower and two – I will be hungry!

I finish up this cardio session and hit the shower. Once I'm clean, refreshed and ready for work, it's time for a very important part of my body transformation goal. It's time to prep food for the day and to eat my first meal!

My kitchen is compact and I have six meals to prepare before I go to work, just like I did yesterday and the day before that. I grab the small saucepan that I always use to cook my brown rice for the day. This has been sitting on the draining board following its wash after I used it last thing last night. The kettle gets filled up and set to boil. While this is doing its thing, I measure out two cups of brown rice and put this in the faithful saucepan.

When the kettle boils, it's my cue to start the rice cooking and get an instant coffee on the go. No milk or sugar, only plain old black coffee on this diet!

While I'm drinking my coffee, I pour 100ml of egg whites into my frying pan and set them cooking with a sprinkle of black pepper and paprika. While the eggs are cooking, I measure out half a cup of rolled oats and a scoop of whey protein powder and put this into a bowl with some water from the kettle.

The eggs are now cooked so I eat them right from the pan. If you've got this much to do every morning before work, any time saving on the washing up is a big help. The egg whites are in and next the oats and protein shake goes down.

It's time to prep my mid-morning meal, my lunch, and my mid-afternoon meal. Four chicken breasts get sliced up and thrown on my griddle with some chilli and garlic. Once these are cooked, the rice is also now ready. The chicken and rice get split into 3 containers and set aside, ready to take to work.

The next thing is to cut a big head of broccoli into florets and put them into a separate container before giving it a quick blast in the microwave. I grab my protein shaker and fill the empty container with a scoop of post workout protein shake. This is all gathered up, and it goes into my food bag. Most people take a single sandwich bag or lunch box to work with them. I take a whole bag and a bunch of containers.

The last part of my morning routine is to wash the dishes I used. I'll need some of these for later in the evening. With the clean-up process complete, it's time to head out to work.

10:30 am comes around pretty quickly, but I'm on a call in the office! I really need to wrap this up because I've got more important things to do. I need to eat!

10:45 am and I finally hang up the call, put my phone on divert and grab my first container of chicken, rice and broccoli out of my bag, I head out of the office into the stairwell, sit on the windowsill and start eating. Out of respect for my work colleagues (no one wants to sit next to the guy who cracks open a plastic container full of chicken and broccoli first thing in the morning) and to also ensure that I could follow my diet plan, I had requested that instead of having a thirty minute lunch break; I had two fifteen minute breaks instead to allow me to get this food in. Once this meal is in, I sit back at my desk and gulp down a big helping of water from my two litre bottle that's always with me.

13:45 pm is my next meal. I go through the same process of finishing a call, taking out my second chicken, rice and broccoli container and head into the stairwell to eat. Back in the office after this meal and back to work.

17:00 pm is the end of my working day and I can hang up my telephone, put my headset back on its charger until tomorrow and once again, head out to the stairwell to eat for the last time at work today. Once I've finished, I will collect all of my things, refill my water bottle and head to the gym to lift some weights followed by another twenty minute, fat burning cardio session.

19:00 pm I add water to the post workout protein powder that I prepared first thing in the morning, shake this up and drink it down. I do this in the car on my way home from the gym and by the time I get home I have finished this shake. It's time for another shower, followed by a bit of computer gaming.

22:00 pm I head to the kitchen, grab my saucepan and set the kettle boiling. I add another half cup of brown rice to the pan, once the kettle is boiled, I add the water to the rice and cooking has started. The brown rice is cooked and I take it off the gas and add a scoop of whey protein powder to it, I then blend this with a hand blender to make a kind of pudding. Because the protein powder is chocolate flavour, this is one of the easiest things that I get to eat every day. Once this is in, I once again wash the dishes I have used so they are ready for me to use first thing tomorrow.

Before bed, I take my shirt off, look in the mirror and hold myself as if I were on stage in front of the judges, just as I've been taught by my posing coach. I look lean and muscular; I see a well-defined set of abs; I see the separation of muscle on my shoulders; I see serratus and obliques. I see the work really paying off, but I want more!

"were getting there," I say out loud.

5:45 am and the familiar sound of the morning alarm brings me out of a deep sleep just like it did yesterday morning and the day before that…

Now is the time to shatter a few common misconceptions and give out some brutally honest advice that needs to be heard by anyone who has struggled to lose weight through dieting before, by making the statement:

"There are no quick fixes or short cuts to lifelong weight management,"

It may sound negative from the outset but once you understand this, stop looking for quick fixes or easy dieting methods and understand that you already have the power to achieve your weight loss goals, but it will take a bit of work upfront and consistent effort, you will have broken down the barriers to entry that hold so many people back from weight loss success and in doing so, you will have made a life changing, positive transformation. This is one of the books many aims. You will see that mind-set plays a huge part in this game.

I'm James and the diary example above was my life while I was dieting for a bodybuilding competition. If this story sounds tough and puts you off wanting to diet for weight loss or any other body transformation, this was kind of my point. Sure this is an extreme example, and it certainly doesn't have to be this way, but the bottom line is that dieting is hard work and if you want to achieve a certain body composition, the result will be a product of your work and commitment.

Anyone that tells you they have an easy way for you to lose weight or get toned, lean or even shredded should be asked the question:

"Easy, compared to what?"

Or

"Easy in what respect?"

The daily, diet and lifestyle diary that I just shared with you would be easy to follow and stick to compared to a daily jog up mount Everest for twenty weeks and it would be very easy if the only food you wanted to eat was chicken, rice and broccoli and you really loved the prep time, washing up and eating on a constant timer, it would be a breeze!

But for the vast majority of people (myself included) this is very inconvenient and unrealistic. This brings me to the point of this book. During the time I spent on this diet, I learned an awful lot, not only what it takes to bring about a decent body transformation in a relatively short time but I learned of nutrition, sustainability, psychological effects (both positive and negative), and these collective lessons, personal experience coupled with my passion for the subject has given me a lot to share.

Sharing my diet knowledge and experience is not the only aim though. I want to help you use this information to change your routine, learn a new subject, actually experiencing a journey to reach a goal. Whether this is dieting or any other matter, it takes time, continued effort, willingness to adapt and learn from any mistakes that you might make.

With this in mind, I also want to offer actionable advice that will help you make smart decisions when it comes to your own diet and lifestyle, allowing you to reach your personal body transformation goals sustainably, in a way that suits you.

There is more than one way to get a great body transformation; some will suit you better than others, so let's find your path!

This guide has all the information that you need to succeed with weight loss, fat loss and body composition change, but I want to offer two solutions. There will be a "level 1" and a "level 2".

Level 1

If you are a total beginner and would like to get started with the basics, you don't want to count calories, do any calculations or work out macros and such. There is a way to do this and still get excellent results with your weight loss plans. Level 1 is also a sound choice if you want to break yourself in gently. You can start here and as you become more familiar with it and you progress, you will find a transition to level 2 pretty smooth and less daunting.

My approach to fitness and diet has always been to keep it simple. I know that if you do the basics right, you can get some amazing results! This means that if you decide to only opt for level 1, there will be no over complicated scientific explanations. I aim to keep this as straight forward as possible.

Level 2

If you have mastered level 1, you can get started with level 2 as a progression. You can also start here if you would like to be more precise from the outset. Level 2 is what I would call a "personal trainers approach".

With the tools and equipment that most of us have available to us, this is the most precise estimate of what your body needs for your weight loss plans. Level 2 will take you through the process that most fitness instructors and serious athletes will follow in order to get the best estimated starting point based on their lifestyle and goals.

There is a fair bit of upfront work with this method, but there is a good overlap of advice from level 1 that can be used and further developed.

I will also end this introduction by reinforcing the fact that this book, like all of my books and guides is based on my personal experience and I believe that the anecdotes I share will be game changing for some readers while others will see them as fluff.

These real-life situations have led me down the path I walk today, have helped me learn valuable lessons and if you can learn these lessons from me, you will get to where you want to be quicker than I ever did and what's more, you will have the knowledge to plan and execute your own diet and lifestyle journey with great success.

I know however that we all process information in different ways, and if these stories are not your thing, you can skip these chapters.

There is a certain mind-set and mental approach to the way we perceive dieting for weight loss that can really help us embrace any changes that we need to make on this journey to success, so before we get into what to eat and when to eat, these will be covered. There are a few pieces to this puzzle,

Everyone has the pieces; it's putting them together in the right order where most of us get stuck. If you want to bring about any change in your life, the first piece of the puzzle is always a shift in mind-set, and dieting for any result is no exception.

"Weight loss" or "Fat loss?" Mind-Set Revelations.

Before we get into the planning and prep, there are a few points that can really help you with the mental side of a successful weight loss and diet venture, so let's start with a game changing mind-set revelation!

A major turning point in mind-set change for the subject of "weight loss" is understanding that the actual goal is "fat loss".

The exclusive use of scales and lbs lost as the measure of success can be misleading and sometimes disheartening because there's a lot more going on.

Most people's idea of weight loss is to "lose their belly", "burn off their love handles" or tighten up their "wobbly bits" and quiet rightly these surplus parts are excess and unwanted body weight, so losing them will cause overall "weight loss".

So why is using the scales and lbs lost so misleading? The simple answer is body composition. If you decide to start a "weight loss" venture, you eat a healthy balanced diet with the right nutrition and you also decide to join a gym, lift some weights and start some form of cardio exercise. You will initially get some "weight loss". This will be in the form of body fat and your body may also retain less water and in general, the systems that your body runs on will work more efficiently.

But after a few weeks, you may stop losing weight. Is something wrong? Has the diet and healthy way of living stopped working? Of course it hasn't. If you are dieting and eating the right foods whilst exercising, you will develop muscle. If you are relying on the scales and lbs lost when you get to this point, it can be disheartening enough to quit and accept that your weight loss venture hasn't worked this time, so it's back to the drawing board to try something new. When in fact this is the point where things are really starting to work!

The holy grail of any "weight loss" goal is not to lose as much weight as possible, but to have more lean muscle than body fat. Once you are on your way to developing muscle and burning body fat, you will find it easier to burn more body fat moving forward.

Using the scales and counting lbs lost is a measure that you can use initially, and every now and again through your fitness journey, but it should not be the number one measure of your success.

I would always advise that if you are setting out to start a "weight-loss diet" that you incorporate some form of resistance and cardio exercise as well. Not only will this be a big help to your overall goal, but it will also keep you strong, healthy and is ultimately responsible for your body shape.

It's common to see people set out to "lose weight" and neglect all that is mentioned in this section. If the only goal is to "lose weight" and body composition is not considered, there is no exercise program in place, there's zero concern about where the weight that's lost comes from, this can cause issues with strength, muscle definition and even posture.

Coming from a bodybuilding background where physique, proportion, balance and symmetry is the goal, it's very apparent to me when someone has achieved an amazing weight loss goal but has neglected to work on body composition on their journey. So from now on, when we use the phrase "weight loss" we really mean "Fat loss and lean muscle development".

Other issues that need to be addressed from the outset are the timescale and goal of the weight-loss diet. If we revisit my diet outlined in the preface, we know that this was an extreme situation for an extreme goal. This was a twenty-week diet and even though twenty weeks sounds like a long time, it's actually a short-term goal in this game. This particular diet was used to reach a temporary result. The mental aspect was brutal, it was expensive; it was all-consuming and all round unsustainable for my set of circumstances, and unless you have a temporary goal like mine back then, there is no reason to be doing a diet of this kind.

Do you set out to "lose this belly", "get rid of these love handles" or "lose these wobbly bits" for a few months only, or do you set out on a weight-loss diet to lose them permanently? Of course you want the permanent fix! So do I. This is why planning for the long term, creating a diet that you can make a part of your life and understanding things like body composition is the way to go for everyone that sets out to achieve this life-changing goal.

You don't need fad diets, weight loss supplements or quick fixes and you don't need to be a human biologist or a nutritional expert to get these results, you just need to know a few basic things and execute them well.

I want to help you diet for weight loss but I also want to help you plan your journey so upon reaching the finish line you will be lean, toned, strong, balanced, knowledgeable and an inspiration to others wanting to walk your path. I want not only to help you lose weight; I want to help you change your body composition; I want to help you lose body fat, tone muscle and I want to give you a solution to do this sustainably so you cannot just change your body, but you can change your lifestyle and take this forward with you far into your future.

Most people call me Jim these days. I've had a long journey in fitness and all that it stands for. I have not only formal qualifications in health and fitness training, but I have a lot of experience and stories to tell that show "blood on the floor" and "against the odds" success and I know these will help many people get to where they want to be when it comes to their personal fitness goals in a fraction of the time that it took me.

Putting all the metaphors aside for now though, the reason for writing this book is based on my experience of the diet and weight loss advice that is rarely talked about and to help anyone that is serious about achieving impressive weight loss results actually get there and stay there. Sure, there are plenty of ways to lose body fat or tone up in a relatively short time, but there is a lot that goes with this that is almost never mentioned.

For example – You see a "before and after" picture on social media, on an advert or any other myriad of platforms that are promoting a diet product or theory and you want a piece of that! This is often the trigger or starting point for a potential weight loss aspirant and a way into the game.

Assuming that this weight loss advert is genuine, it doesn't show you the truth. The person in the picture or video had a lot more going on than whatever product or idea is being pushed.

Whether this success story used a certain product or followed a certain type of diet plan, they would not have arrived at this success without commitment, consistency, a big change in lifestyle, a certain amount of knowledge and sacrifice to some extent.

It's my aim to give you all the tools that you need to actually be one of these diet and weight loss success stories and to do it in the best way for your specific set of circumstances.

4 proven steps for successful diet creation TLDR

There are some marvellous stories of body transformations and weight loss success from a myriad of personalities, and if these are documented on any media platform, the same question is always asked -

"What's the secret?"

Of course, we would always love to hear that it's something weird, wonderful and most importantly, quick and easy.

It would be amazing to think that eating blueberries under a full moon at midnight changing nothing else in our lives would cause a jaw dropping body transformation.

Or drinking a "proprietary blend" shake of "Dr six packs chocolate flavour muscle shake dust", would have us lean, muscular and tanned in just two short weeks.

Deep down we all know this is not a reality but most of us at some point will be drawn into the idea that there is another way that's more fun, quicker and easier than the reality.

The reality however is always going to be the true answer to success, and it really is pretty simple, the only tricky part is commitment.

Aside from leaving behind any hype around weight loss shortcuts, diet methods and magic pills that may draw you in, there are only four steps that you need to take for a guaranteed body transformation success story of your own.

We will cover this in a lot more detail and by the time you have finished the book, you will have you're your very own diet plan and be ready to go! But here is the reality and a TLDR ("Too long didn't read") for the rest of the book.

Step 1 – Get a goal

We all set out on this journey to achieve something. The clearer you can make your goal, the better. If you decide that your goal is to "lose weight", that's good, but you can do better. The more specific that you can be, the more connected you will be with your goal. If your goal is too general, it's easier to lose track of. To get a more specific version of a general "weight loss goal", ask questions like –

- How much weight do I want to lose?
- Why do I want to do this?
- What is my timescale for this amount of weight loss?

So a goal that was originally just to "lose weight" could become something like "Lose 60lbs of body fat to run the Boston half marathon in September"... Oh yeah, I have always advised that you should also be ambitious when creating your goals, everyone is capable of achieving a lot more than they think they are!

Step 2 – Do a food diary for 2 weeks

This step is extremely valuable. It's true to say that you don't need to know what you were eating if you decide to draw a line in the sand and start a completely new lifestyle in the diet and nutritional department. I know that many people who have had great success with their body transformation didn't do this, but it is a wholly worthwhile process as you will learn so much about yourself, your habits and be able to pinpoint areas of your lifestyle where you can make quick wins for exponentially positive progress.

So if you want the edge over everyone else, do a food diary! This is what you do-

- Start at the beginning of a week and make sure you have at least 2 weeks of "normal life" ahead of you, no holidays, no events, etc.
- Write down everything that you eat and drink every day. EVERYTHING.
- With this information and a bit of knowledge of food types and nutrition, you will see exactly what you are doing right and what you are doing wrong.

Step 3 – Do the basics and do them well

You know what you want to achieve, now you need a good plan that aligns. This is where it can go wrong for many people. With the subject of weight loss in particular, there are a lot of ways to get the same result so if you set out to find "the best" weight loss plan, it's likely that your search will end in confusion or worse yet, it will never end.

A lot of weight loss diets and body transformation plans run from a subset of theories or lifestyle changes, but if you look closely, they will all be rooted in and built from basic food nutrition knowledge.

On the surface, you may see two diet plans that preach polar opposite views, but both claim to be the "best diet for weight loss" but if you look a bit deeper, you will probably see some similarities. A quick example of this is a "Vegan diet for weight loss" vs an "exclusively carnivorous diet for weight loss". You will see that they both depend on the following values.

- Don't eat refined sugar
- Eat whole foods
- Don't eat processed foods
- Don't eat too much
- Do some exercise

For the creation of your weight loss plan, the above list is solid. These are the basic rules for any diet plan, weight loss or otherwise. To guarantee our success, however, we need to learn how to use these rules to turn our goals into achievements. So instead of looking for the answers in diet methods or supplements, take these points with plenty of water.

Step 4 – Stick with it and make adjustments when you need to

If you just sold your cow for some magic beans, or maybe some of that "chocolate flavour muscle dust", and you expect to wake up the next morning to see a huge beanstalk has grown or wake up to see that the muscle dust has actually worked, you will probably be disappointed.

We don't live in a fairy tale, but if you find some magic beans or muscle dust that works, please give me a shout!

All joking aside, the only way that anyone will earn results is to stick with it, not only that but always keep adjusting things as you progress. It is really rare to get things right on the first attempt. The longer your journey is, and the more consistently you seek improvements, the better your results will be. So keep an open mind, remember your goal, recognise your mistakes, learn from them and learn about yourself.

The real secret to weight loss and world class body transformations can never be attributed to a single supplement, method of dieting, or a single food type. There are no secrets in this game, there's just knowledge and commitment.

What's the best diet? It's a learning process

So what's the best diet to follow to get this long term, sustainable fat loss and body composition change? The truth is that there are many ways to do this! The perfect diet for you hinges on a few things:

- What you and your set of circumstances can handle
- Your knowledge of food and how your body deals with it
- Your drive to make it happen.

What can you handle?

To outline this point with an extreme example, let's imagine that you are a raw vegan and you want to diet for fat loss (Yes it is possible for a raw vegan to have excess fat stores). You read an article on someone who ate organ meat and saturated fats exclusively to lose all of their excess body fat and not only build a superb physique but build impressive physical strength to boot.

If you were a raw vegan, and this is the exact result that you wanted to achieve. I very much doubt that this type of diet is something that you would try, and even if you tried it, what are the odds that you could maintain this for a lifetime, given the nutritional situation that you currently found yourself in?

It's not just the type of food that has a bearing on whether you can handle a certain diet, there are other factors to consider. Sticking with this example, if "raw" food is not cooked, and you are used to not cooking, this will make a big difference in food prep, so you would have to adjust for this.

If you have been a raw vegan for a long time, your body might not react too well to cooked meat products and animal fats, and the all-important, mental aspect of the food you eat can sometimes have the biggest bearing in whether or not you can handle a change.

Why are you on a vegan diet in the first place? Is it because animal welfare is your driving force? If this is the case, how do you bring yourself to brush this under the carpet? If you just prefer to eat raw, plant based food, why would you switch to food that you didn't like?

We can also flip this around to make a more realistic example. Let's imagine that you are very overweight, out of shape, and have eaten whatever you wanted, whenever you wanted, never really had an interest in nutrition or cooking and this has been your approach for your entire life and now you want to change.

You watch a YouTube video on raw vegan bodybuilders and you decide that this is the result that you want, so you set out on a raw vegan diet.

Given your history, this would be very challenging as first you would need to learn a lot about nutrition, you would have to get used to meal prep, you would have to be a lot more organised and you would have to actually like the food you were eating and the lifestyle that comes with this to make it sustainable.

If you had been used to eating pizza, takeaways, going out to restaurants, never had an interest in looking at food labels, never needed to plan and prep your meals, this would be a huge undertaking. The mental robustness needed for this type of change would be challenge enough alone without even considering the physical side of it.

Whenever you change an aspect of your diet, there will be challenges. The trick to sustainability and long term success is to minimise these challenges and overcome them one at a time. This is a measured approach to the lifestyle change and in my experience, it is more successful than making a full lifestyle change overnight, like the examples mentioned here.

It is however possible to draw a line in the sand and make a drastic change to your diet and lifestyle overnight, but this can be really stressful and it has greater scope for disaster this way.

So when it comes to changing your diet for weight loss, one of the biggest questions that most people don't ask before they start is:

"What level of change can I handle?"

Your knowledge of food and how your body deals with it.

Since my early teens, when I first set out to achieve a fitness goal, I knew that protein repairs muscle and helps you grow; I knew that carbohydrates give you energy, water helps to transport the nutrients around your body, so you need plenty of that, and I knew that too much chocolate will make you fat.

This is very basic knowledge, but over the years I've not stopped learning about these "rules". I've looked into this more and more as my ever increasingly ambitious fitness goals dictated, and this knowledge has enabled me to make good decisions when it comes to the food I will eat on a daily basis - my diet.

Knowledge is power! But as mentioned earlier, you don't have to be a guru in nutrition and systems of the human body to achieve significant results in diet and weight loss. The best way to approach this is to do it in the same way that you would when incorporating dietary changes into your lifestyle; you should overcome each challenge as it presents itself.

I started off by knowing the basics about nutrition and taking what I learned, putting it into practice and then asking questions about the basics. For example, we know that protein builds and repairs muscle, but what foods have the best protein source for my fitness goals? This is another step in the right direction in understanding nutrition, and it builds on what we already know.

Another example is that we know that too much chocolate will make us fat. But why? After asking this question it turns out that it's not actually the chocolate that's the big problem, it's the refined sugar in the chocolate that's going to cause us issues. Knowing this information gives us two more questions to ask –

"Why is refined sugar so bad?"

And

"What other foods could be hiding refined sugar?"

Why is refined sugar so bad? Asking this question will lead you down the road of how your body processes the types of food you put into it, you will learn about hormones in the human body and how you can help them to help you. You will learn to appreciate and understand that the calories you fuel your body with can be really useful or totally useless.

What other foods could be hiding refined sugar? If this is the first time you are hearing about hidden refined sugars in foods and you start looking, you will probably be extremely shocked at what you find and this will lead you to yet more questions.

It's worth mentioning here that "adding to your knowledge" may mean that you change your standing on something based on your own experience or new knowledge that you have gained. An example of this in my personal journey was that when I started out on a muscle building goal, I totally neglected my complex carbohydrate intake and focused only on the protein intake in my diet, because based on my basic knowledge, I believed that carbohydrates only gave me energy and had no part to play in building muscle mass.

After some study, and asking "why am I not growing like I should be?" and then seeking the knowledge from bodybuilders that were getting results from their diets, I found that this was not the case so I had to change my outlook on complex carbohydrates completely! Complex carbohydrates became my best friends!

But if we look at this knowledge gathering and understanding as a long-term goal as we did with the changes made to diet, the point is not to know and learn everything overnight. The point is to start with a solid, basic foundation and then add more progress over time as you evolve with your diet, lifestyle and fitness success.

This is how your journey of knowledge and nutritional understanding should work. It's also very important to appreciate that other people will follow a different road and connect with diet and nutrition practices that you don't agree with, but if these people can find long-term, sustainable diet success in their way, then it works for them and they should be congratulated!

Always be open-minded, ask "why?" and "how?".

Your drive to make it happen.

If you have a good enough reason to diet for weight loss or any other fitness result, you will overcome the tough challenges, you will deal with more of these at the same time and when it comes to knowledge and learning about nutrition, this will be an easier task too.

There is a lot to be said about motivation and the bearing this has on your chances of success and you will know all about that if you found your way here after reading my previous book *"Fitness & Exercise Motivation"*.

I truly believe that if you find your reason and it is good enough to motivate you as an individual, you can guarantee your success in any fitness venture.

No one has an easy time when starting out on a body transformation, and for the total beginner, the challenges are all the more challenging. I've never heard of a weight loss or body transformation story that didn't have its fair share of setbacks.

The truth is that it's never a straight road and one of the major skills to work on and master is the skill to pick yourself up when you fall down, learn from your mistakes and carry on towards your goal. If you can do this while using the rest of the information in this book, there is no reason you won't find complete success from your efforts.

When, not "if" you get knocked down, because you will get knocked down, get up, understand what put you down and look out for the same obstacle in the future. You will be better equipped to deal with it next time it pops up.

The calorie deficit vs other diet ideas.

The calorie deficit, (eating fewer calories than you use for energy) for the goal of weight loss is considered by an increasingly growing number of people to be an "old school idea". But the bottom line is that it works, and it always will if you understand and practice the basics.

It really is a simple concept, but the reason that this idea is misunderstood is that there are actually several parts to eating in a calorie deficit to reduce body fat percentage.

The well-known term:

> *"Calories in vs calories out,"*

Is fairly accurate, but if you want to achieve an effective body composition change that also delivers a healthy, strong and efficient body, a more accurate term should be:

> *"Useful calories in vs calories out consistently,"*

The quality of the calories in

The amount of calories or energy that you put into your body on a daily basis is an important factor, but if those calories come from high energy, low-quality foods, you won't be fuelling your body correctly. You won't be giving it what it needs to work efficiently. A couple of slices of pepperoni pizza could be 500 calories, but a chicken breast, a jacket potato and a portion of broccoli could also be 500 calories. Which 500 calorie meal is the best fuel for your body?

Yes, it's the chicken and potato option. I can also tell you that you will get more food on your plate with 500 calories worth of chicken breast and jacket potato than you would with 500 calories of pepperoni pizza.

Calories out

This is the amount of energy you burn. Your body does actually burn a certain amount of calories just by being alive. This is called your "Basal metabolic rate" or "BMR". This amount depends on your current condition, but more on that later.

With this in mind, it is possible to lose weight by eating fewer calories than you burn by sitting on a sofa all day, but it's a far more healthy option to add in an exercise routine to get the most value from your efforts.

If you are eating good, quality calories at a deficit and you are also working out regularly, you will stimulate the systems in your body that burn calories as part of your daily life which will make your body more efficient and ultimately get you to where you want to be with your goals in a shorter time.

Consistency

We all use the measure of a single day for calories in vs calories out and diet plans in general. This is solid as there's always a start and finish, and by working one day at a time, it fits into most people's routines and is easy to break down into bite-size chunks.

It's the consistency that brings all of this together. If you are not consistent with maintaining a calorie deficit over a sustained period, you will have very little or even zero weight loss results. Ideally every day's calorie intake needs to be at a deficit until you have a good routine with meal prep, eating, exercise and you are happy with your current weight. Then things can be reassessed, goals can be updated and so on.

So what's the difference between using a calorie deficit and focusing on where those calories come from diet and other popular diet ideas and theories that don't use calorie counting, and why would you decide to follow another method?

If you completely ignore the type's foods that you eat, you eat all the bad stuff, pizza, ice cream, chocolate and just eat at a calorie deficit. Guess what?

You will lose weight. But among other disadvantages, you won't feel your best and you will be hungry. Why? The simple answer to this is that if you eat low quality, fast burning sugars/ carbohydrates, you will be empty quicker.

With so many fad diets, diet gurus, contradicting information and in-depth theories and ideas out there, it's easy to forget some fundamental facts at the very foundation of anyone's ability to burn excess body fat. The bottom line is that if you want to lose body fat, you have to use more calories than you are putting in.

I've read articles, watched videos of fitness professionals and seen the idea banded around that you can lose weight and burn body fat without the need of a calorie deficit and this is not helpful advice for anyone getting into this game.

There are no (safe) supplements or pills that help you lose body fat without the need of a calorie deficit.

The more wholesome the food that you eat is, the lower in calories to weight ratio and higher in useful nutritional value that food will be. So you need to eat a bigger volume of chicken breast, broccoli and rice to get the same amount of calories from a few slices of peperoni pizza.

On top of this, the benefit of eating the chicken, rice and broccoli vs the pizza is also that the peperoni pizza will have minimal useful nutrition for your body to use.

If you put these two meals in front of most people and asked them which is the best for your body, I would imagine that the majority, if not all, would say that the chicken and rice wins. But I would also bet that a lot would not know exactly why. This is what we will discuss in the next section.

To finish off this section, I would like to add that other diet methods and theories are also effective and can be used alongside a calorie deficit and whole, quality food approach but this should be your first priority.

Understand the calorie deficit and get to know the quality levels of foods before you venture into things like fasting, keto, paleo etc.

Level 1 - Four steps to weight loss & diet success

It's very common when you hear the word "diet" to immediately think "Weight loss". The singular word diet means;

> *"The food you eat on a daily basis,"*

I want to invite you into this way of thinking. Whether you like it or not, the food that you put into your body is the "Diet that you are on". Everybody is on a diet of some kind. Some people may be on a "see food" diet ("if I see it, I'll eat it"), some may be on a vegetarian diet, some may be on a dairy-free diet, and the list goes on.

If you can put all the food, you eat or even encounter into a category, and understand how these categories of food can benefit your body and ultimately your fitness goal, you'll be on track to make the best choices.

One of the primary aims of this guide is to help you understand the properties of different foods simplistically, and this is all the knowledge that anyone needs to create their own weight-loss diet and make the right food choices.

For sustainable fat loss and body composition changes that relate to diet and nutrition, there are only really four areas that you need to understand and implement. So before you get caught up in ketogenic, Atkins, fasting, 4:1, paleo, or anything like this that resembles a "method" of dieting, start here!

This is for everyone because if you can understand the foods you fuel your body with and what effects they have on you as an individual, you will be able to make your own informed decisions about any dieting method and establish whether this is the right path for you.

In this section, we will look at these all important, four areas in a step-by-step manner in priority order.

Step - #1 Know the food

Every type of food is simply energy. Anything that is edible for us humans is a form of energy. The single measure of this energy that we use is called a calorie.

As well as an amount of calories (energy) in a certain amount of food, there are also a different set of properties in these foods too (these are known as "macronutrients" or "Macros"), but we don't really need to know what these are on a molecular level right now, you can look into that later as your journey gets more advanced if you really want to.

Some foods have more energy per pound than others, and some foods have far more useful properties too. The quality of the properties in the food that you eat can help your body to develop and have a huge influence in steering you toward your fitness and body transformation goal.

For sensible food choices, your priority is to look for food that is made up of the best, most useful properties and then look to the amount of energy that these foods offer as the next step.

Although there are many approaches to nutrition and diet for weight loss and there is a lot more going on with every type of food than a single benefit to the human body, for the purpose of this level 1 section and creating your first long-term, sustainable diet plan, we will focus on 5 "food types".

Every food will not fit directly into one of these "food types" but the aim of this is to be able to match every food choice that you make with one of these "food types" based on the most abundant property of that food.

The 5 food types that we will focus on are: Protein, Fat, Complex carbohydrates, Fibrous goodness and "treats and cheats".

Food types:

Protein – This energy source is the building blocks. Protein is used to build and repair our body and plays a vital part in body composition change. Some good examples of this food type include lean cuts of meat, poultry and white fish.

Fats – Energy dense or calorie dense nutrition that helps regulate energy storage and certain vitamins. Fat also helps your body to function correctly. Some good examples of this food type include nuts, avocado, coconut oil, quality cheese.

Complex carbohydrates – Foods that your body prefers to use for energy. This energy is slow release, can be stored in the muscles for later use, and helps to keep you fuller for longer. Some good examples of this food type include: Oats, Brown rice, Brown pasta, Granary bread, beans.

Fibrous goodness – Foods that are a low source of energy or low in calories, so foods of this type are ideal for filling up on. These foods are also a source of vitamins, minerals, and fibre. Some good examples of this food type include Broccoli, asparagus, Kale, green beans and green salad foods.

Treats and cheats – Foods that are high in energy or calorie dense, but are made up of low quality properties. These foods can cause systems in the body to be less efficient and are most likely to be responsible for excess weight gain and fat storage. Some good examples of this food type include Cakes, pastries and chocolate, potato chips, sugary drinks, Fast food and takeaway food in general.

Step #2 Know the energy of the properties –

"To lose weight, I must eat fewer calories!". It has always been a frustration of mine when a beginner to weight loss decides that their first port of call must be to reduce the energy intake of their food. As a reminder - eating fewer calories means reducing the amount of energy that you put into your body.

While this is true to a certain extent and it may work, I believe that this is far from optimal. By this way of thinking, it would not matter where the calories came from and the properties or macros that the foods I ate were made up of. I could, by this theory, decide to eat 2500 calories of orange flavour sherbet every day and this would be just fine.

If you know the properties of the energy or if you know what the calories you are eating do for your body, you will have a far better chance of reaching your fitness or weight loss goals as you will give your body the right fuel to function to its optimum.

The bottom line is that your body needs calories not only to develop, but it needs calories to function. Every system that your body runs on (and there are a lot of these) depends on this energy, too. So if you have to give it calories, you may as well give it quality calories. And orange flavour sherbet is not a quality calorie.

Protein – Has 4 calories per gram

Fat – Has 9 calories per gram

Complex carbohydrate – Has 4 calories per gram

Fibrous goodness – For this guide, calories from foods that fit this type are negligible as the benefits outweigh the content.

Treats and cheats – Foods that fit into this type are calorie dense and/ or have low or even zero useful properties. Calories from these foods are not useful for development and nutritionally empty. You may have heard the term "empty calories" to describe foods of this type.

As you can see, quality complex carbs and protein are far less energy dense than quality fats that have over double the calories per gram, and this has some influence when it comes to our next point. But for now, this is just a point that is worth taking a note on.

How much energy does your body need every day? This is a question that cannot be answered definitively for the reason that most questions of this nature in the diet and nutrition game can't –

"everybody is different!"

The best approach is to start with the generic, recommended daily intake set by the authorities in this field. This is –

>2500 calories per day for a male
>
>&
>
>2000 calories per day for a female

There are several different ways of arriving at a starting point and they will all give you different figures. But this is a sound choice. If you are eating quality energy, meaning an amount of quality protein, complex carbs and fat to the tune of 2000/ 2500 calories per day, and you have not done this before, you will soon know whether you need to adjust for your lifestyle and your unique set of circumstances.

We will talk about this later, as this is part of the progression. This figure will be too high for some and too low for others but as we already know, this is a learning process for everyone and every journey needs a start. And with that, we are ready for step #3.

Step #3 – Ratios

There is much discussion about the ratios of the food types or "macros" that you should eat, and this varies massively from nutrition coach to nutrition coach.

There are advocates for high fat, high protein and zero carbs, there are weight-loss diet theories that push zero fat and high protein. I have even heard of a water only diet!... But we are not going there! ☺

I think that in this day and age, if you look for a diet that favours a certain food type, you will find one that's dedicated to it. When it comes to ratios of these food types, there is a certain aspect of "what can you handle" and "what are your beliefs" discussed in a previous chapter, and this may set you on a different path.

This guide, however, is all about having a balanced and measured approach to weight loss diets, and if you are willing to embrace this method, this is the ratio of food types that I would recommend starting out with.

Calories from complex carbs – 40%

Calories from proteins – 40%

Calories from fats – 20%

So your plate should look like this –

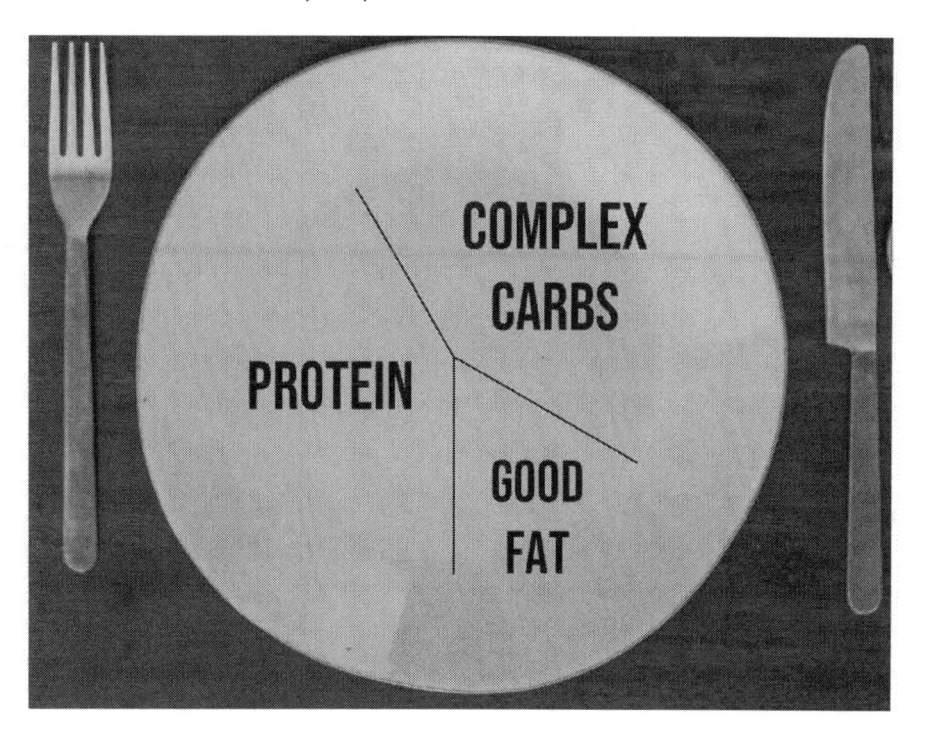

COMPLEX CARBS

PROTEIN

GOOD FAT

Of course, this can be tweaked in favour of one food type over the other in terms of percentage but here's the theory behind this food type ratio –

- 40% carbs - If we assume that complex carbohydrates are our body's favoured form of energy and they have 4 calories per gram, we can eat a bigger quantity of this food type, meaning that we will feel full up. Also, in the early stages of our weight loss venture, there is less risk of hitting a calorie surplus and more margin for error if our portion sizes are not spot on.

- 40% protein – More protein means more repair and recovery. If we are also exercising alongside this diet (which I highly recommend, more on that later too), we will need the protein. More lean muscle means more energy burned at rest, so more opportunity to burn away excess body fat.

- 20% fat – We know that quality fat is a useful food type, but we also know that it's the most calorie dense food type by having over double the amount of calories per gram. This means it makes sense to keep it in check by limiting it by 50% of the other two food types. If we ate the same amount of fat in grams as we did carbs or protein, we would be more than doubling our calorie or energy intake. This would lead to a calorie surplus and could be responsible for excess weight gain.

With the food type "fibrous goodness", you can add these to every meal as they do not have a significant calorie content to impact you negatively. So add foods from this category to bulk out your plate if it looks a bit sparse. Remember, these foods are rich in vitamins and fibre.

Where does the food type "Treats & cheats" fit into the ratio? In short, and to be brutally honest, this food type has no place in a weight-loss diet. But as a lover of pizza, cheeseburgers and slabs of milk chocolate and also as someone who has cut these out of my life completely for long periods of time in the past, I can tell you that the world is not the same without them.

I can also tell you that if you use these foods as treats and allow yourself to disregard all rules during one meal per week, your favourite foods that are firmly in the "treats and cheats" category have never tasted so good!

The golden rule with foods in the treats and cheats category is that you have to see them as occasional treats and not part of your diet. But the bottom line here is that the less you have of this type of food, the better your results will be.

So too much of foods on the treats and cheats list will make you gain excess weight, but too much of any type of food can cause excess weight gain which leads us neatly onto step #4

Step #4 – Portion control

Counting calories and understanding the amount of energy that makes up your meals is the way to do this, but to get it right takes a bit more in-depth working out and planning. This is a level 2 exercise that will be covered later.

Eating too much of any food type can make you gain excess body fat. Why? Because you are giving yourself more fuel than you can use, and the result is stored body fat.

Portion control is extremely important, and there are many ways in which to approach this step. As it is with most other subjects, the more effort that you put into understanding and implementing portion control, the better your results will be.

Portion control ties all the other steps together, and it can be the deciding factor whether you earn your weight loss results or not.

There are ways to make this a bit simpler than it has to be but again, the bottom line is, the more effort that you put into understanding the serving size for each food type upfront, the better your results will be and quicker they will show up.

The following steps may sound like a bit of a chore, but it is an essential part of understanding portion control and will go a long way towards improving your general knowledge of nutrition and helping you identify and adjust your diet when it comes to it.

You may already have some digital kitchen scales. If not, these are widely available and you can pick them up pretty inexpensively these days, so grab a set of these. They are a valuable piece of kit. You should also pick up some measuring cups if you do not own these already. You can get away with just a ¼ cup but having a ½ cup and a 1 cup is also handy.

The best way to approach this is to:

- Take the foods you eat regularly or the foods you plan to get into your diet after reading this guide and first, establish what type of food this is
- Establish how many calories are in a single gram.
- Weigh out the amount that you need, then find a measuring cup or container that this will fit into.
- Once you have done this for food that you will eat regularly, you can just fill that container up for 1 serving and no need to weigh again! Eventually, you will be able to accurately "eyeball" portion size.

Some real-life examples of this that I have used for years are that every day at breakfast time, I use a ½ cup to scoop out my dry rolled oats. I know that this food type is my carbs, and I know that it is about 150 calories. Originally I measured this out on a food scale, but off the top of my head I don't know how many grams this is, but the important thing is that I know how much energy in carbohydrates is going in. I've done this so much now, that I can probably just pour the oats directly into a bowl and pretty much get it right by eyeballing it.

Another example is almonds. I love almonds as a snack, but I know that the food type is mainly fat (a more dense energy) so portion control needs to be a bit tighter here. Originally I would have weighed these out, but since finding the ¼ cup, I don't need the scale, it's just a simple scoop and that's my 200 calories from fat.

If you can understand, practice and master these four principals, you will find success in a body transformation goal.

Diet for weight loss and body composition change is a learning process, it's like any other activity or interest, the more you practise, the more effort that you put in, the better you will get, the easier it will seem and ultimately, the more impressive your end results will be.

In summary:

- Understand the food that you are eating. Take an interest in what makes up the food and learn to identify which type it best fits.
- Understand that fats are made up of far more energy than proteins and carbs
- Learn to identify the ratios of proteins, complex carbs and fats in your meals
- Get to grips with portion control. Dedicate some time upfront to familiarise yourself with what different food types and their properties look like when they are actually on a plate.

Of which food labels?

Food labels can be fairly confusing and as far as my experience goes, I wasn't ever taught about food labels and the understanding of food labels seems to be assumed by many people.

I was one of these people for a long time too, and as far as I was concerned, a food label shows the amount of protein, carbs, fats and sugars so you can make an informed decision on whether the food is a good or bad choice.

This is ok, and you can get by on it, but there's another way to look at labels that simplifies it, brings more clarity and should be a bit of a revelation to most.

So with this in mind, this is a simple way to get big value out of the understanding of food labels.

There are three factors that you should consider that can make a big difference to your understanding.

- The quality of the food based on the ingredients list.
- The "of which" phrase.
- The calories per portion.

The quality of the food based on the ingredients list

The first thing to do is to consider what the actual food is. Is it a snack bar made up of pure fruit with no additional ingredients, is it a protein powder, is it a breakfast cereal? It could be anything that comes in a packet.

Let's stick to two examples. We'll pick a breakfast cereal and a natural fruit snack bar.

If you look at the natural fruit snack bar and the ingredients lists a selection of nothing but fruit and no additives like golden syrup, maltodextrin, gelling agents and any numbers that follows an "E", you know that this is a quality, natural product.

There are plenty of snack bars out there that pitch themselves as being a healthy alternative, but I'm always shocked when I look at the ingredients of most. So if this is your thing, go out and check the food labels after you read this section, you'll no doubt see what I mean.

Breakfast cereal is also another minefield for misinformation. A healthy option is often marketed as "low fat". The big "low fat" sticker on the healthy looking, organic packet can be a very true statement which is enough to get it to the checkout and into the cupboards of us consumers, but if you look at the food label and understand what you are looking at, you'll see that this is a high in sugar, low-quality food that will not help us with our fitness goals.

So the first thing to do is to look at the ingredients part. Is the food in this pack, can or box made of quality ingredients or are there ingredients on this list, things that should not be there, you don't know what they are or is there a phrase that says "proprietary blend".

The last point to make on the ingredients list is that the list starts with the most abundant ingredient and follows to the least. So if you see a food and its first ingredient is "sugar", you know that this is not great at all. If your packet has the first ingredients as "chicken breast" for example, you know you are eating something that's going to give your body some quality fuel.

The "of which" phrase

Once you have determined whether the food in the pack is a good quality food, the next thing to look at is the "Nutrition panel". On this panel, you will see the amounts of "food types" listed. This will be in weight per 100g and / or per serving. This panel will also tell you how many overall calories there are in this 100grams and also a single serving.

The nutrition panel will show you the Fat, carbohydrates, fibre, protein and salt as standard but there should also be two extra fields that start with "of Which".

- Of which saturates
- Of which sugars

Of which saturates should be listed directly underneath the "fat" content, as this is a continuation of the fat content. It means that of the total amount of fat in this product, there is this amount of saturated fat. Of which sugars is the same thing but for the carbohydrates value on the nutrition label.

An example of this - If the amount of fat is listed as 30.8g per 100g and the "of which saturates" is listed underneath as 7.7g. It means that of the 30.8g, 7.7g is saturated fat. This is the same for the "of which sugars" in relation to the carbohydrates.

It's listed like this because saturated fats are considered to be the unhealthy fats, and sugars are considered to be the unhealthy or unuseful carbohydrates.

One caveat of this is that if the ingredients list is a quality one (made up of real, whole foods), the "of which sugars" might be fairly high.

This is why I mentioned the natural fruit snack bar earlier as this makes the point nicely; the "of which sugars" might be high, but it is a quality food and can be good to use right before an exercise session or as part of your regular diet.

With the rest of the information in the book, this should really help you make good decisions and identify the quality of each food you plan to eat that has a label.

The calories per portion

This one is explained in the chapter "A calorie deficit vs other diet ideas" but here's a tip for calories in relation to food labels. With most food labels, we are actually told how many calories are in a 100gs of that food and we are also given a recommended "portion size" too.

The recommended portion size will either be in "per unit". The natural fruit bar will display as "per bar" and have the list on the nutrition label underneath. This is really handy, as you know exactly what you are getting with each bar.

The breakfast cereal and products that come without obvious serving portions will display as a measure in grams. If you are not familiar with the weight of a food of this type, you can easily over eat.

Using scoops and kitchen scales is also covered in another chapter too, but if you've never measured out a recommended portion size before, you might be surprised at what a suggested, single serving looks like. Have a go at this, it's an eye-opening exercise, especially with a lot of popular brands of breakfast cereal.

Meal prep and "one pot cooking"

Once you have your food planned, you've been shopping and are ready to start a new week of your healthy diet, the next step is to prep and cook.

Knowing how much of which types of food to eat is one thing but a critical factor in a long term weight loss success story that is often overlooked is knowing what to do with that food.

So far we've covered the different food types that make up your diet, but how do you turn the theory into a practical, actionable exercise and how does it fit into your average day?

Meal prepping and learning how to cook is one of the best quality of life skills that you can develop when it comes to nutrition and diet for weight loss in particular. If you know how to make tasty, exciting meals that give you all the right nutrients, you will not only have an easier time, but it will be fun!

One of the best ways to keep thing fresh, try new ideas, develop your cooking skills, nutritional knowledge and eventually find some healthy recipes that you love is to try a new recipe every week. In the workbook that acts as a companion guide to this book, there is a page dedicated to exactly this on every new week that you progress to, so be sure to take advantage of this.

The longer that you stick to learning a new recipe per week, the more your recipe library will grow and before long, you'll be able to turn your hand to plenty of healthy food options in the kitchen.

If you do decide to do this, a recipe doesn't have to be a main meal; it could be a snack, like homemade protein bars or a sweet desert option like a fruit flan or diet cookies. Do some research, you will probably be surprised at the healthy alternatives to favourites that you can create for yourself.

and it may feel a bit of a chore at first but the more you do it, the quicker and more efficient you will become at the process.

Daily food prep

Keeping a freezer, fridge and cupboard full of prepped food is great for a longer game such as a week or month but daily food prep is a slightly different type of food prep that leans heavily on this.

A solid diet plan will have set meals with set amounts of nutrients in each meal planned on a daily basis. This means that there will be a certain amount of prep work on a daily basis for most people. Everyone has a different set of daily life commitments and I would venture a guess that a lot of cooking and meal prep doesn't feature heavily in most people's circumstances.

If every meal that you are planning to eat on any day is ready and waiting exactly when you need it, you are winning the battle so make sure this happens. The best way to get a handle on this is to make your first daily job your meal prep for the day ahead.

Obviously, this prep will vary greatly from person to person. If you are leaving the house at 08:00 and won't be back until 20:00, you will need to be a bit more on the ball. Think about everything that you need to eat from the moment you leave until the moment you get home. Are you able to pick up the food that you have on your diet from a shop, or do you need to prep everything before you leave? Look back at the chapter "It works, but it doesn't have to be this way" to get an idea of the mind set of prepping. Again, I will mention that this example is a very extreme way of dealing with food prep but the principals are the same and there are definitely some good takeaways in the account.

The same can be said about daily food prep as can be said about food prep in general, the more you practice it, the quicker and more efficient you will become at getting the job done.

As mentioned earlier, batch cooking and one pot cooking are super convenient cooking and food prep practices that I would highly recommend having a go at and getting to grips with. So here are some tips

Tips for batch cooking and prep

- Invest in freezer bags, tin foil rolls/ trays and plastic containers

Once you make a big pot of food that will serve you for several meals, make it even easier for future meal times by dividing it up into single serving portions, putting it in a container, wrapping it in foil or filling freezer bags.

By having ready-made, single serving portions to hand, you will save lots of time and effort and you'll become really efficient with your diet. If you can get containers that are stackable, even better for storage.

A point to note about freezing batch cooked meals and to further reinforce the benefit of ready-made, single serving portions is that if you freeze a full batch cooked meal as a whole, you will have to defrost it as a whole and this can really take from your efficiency.

The same thing goes for prep. If you buy fresh food in bulk such as steak mince or chicken breast, you should separate the portions before freezing so when it comes to cooking, you don't just have a 5kg block of chicken breast to work with.

- **Use a slow cooker or soup maker**

Slow cookers and soup makers are great for batch cooking and are really suited to meals like casseroles, chilli and more obviously, soups.

Batch cooking these types of meals is not only fairly quick and easy but you also have great flexibility for creativity. You can decide what foods you want in a soup, stew or casserole based on your diet plans and just throw it in to make a one pot meal. More on one pot cooking later though!

- **Organise your food storage**

If your fridge, freezer, food cupboards and pantry are all organised, you will be organised when it comes to cooking, food prep, creating your shopping list and it will probably help you more than you think with your diet plans in general.

Tidy your freezer draws and organise the storage by using stackable containers containing the same meals together, having a place for fresh veg, meat and fruit. You can also do this for your fridge, have a dairy section, a greens section and a "Meals ready to go" section.

Everyone will eventually fall into their own rhythm with this type of thing and it all depends on the individual so these are some ideas if this is a new concept.

Tips for one pot cooking

- **Get a big metal or cast iron pan with a lid**

One pot cooking is one of my preferred cooking methods, not only because it saves on the washing up or that it works well with batch cooking, but it's an incredibly efficient way to make some really tasty meals!

The first thing you need to get if you are going to get into this cooking method is a good pot. You should look for a quality cast iron, non-stick or metal pot that's big and deep. The pot should also be usable on gas, electric hobs, be oven proof and have a lid.

A good pan can be expensive but this will last you a lifetime and in my opinion, it's worth the investment. At the time of writing, I have a mid-range pot that I've been using most days for over ten years and it's still going strong.

A good pan as mentioned above is extremely versatile as it can be used as a frying pan, saucepan, baking tray and even a steamer.

- **Build the flavours in a single pot**

Whatever recipe you cook as a one pot meal, the cooking process will normally go through a set of stages. You will tend to use the pot slightly differently in each stage. The first stage is normally to use the pot as if it were a frying pan to fry over gas, brown or soften ingredients.

If I were making a chilli, I would fry onions in a little butter or oil, once these were slightly brown, I would then push the onions to one side of the pan, add the steak mince and brown this. Part way through the mince browning, I would mix the onions in to stop them burning.

With the browning out of the way, it's time to add the spices, herbs and flavourings, once this is mixed in, the next stage is to use the pot as if it were a saucepan. Staying with the chilli example, I would add tinned tomatoes, kidney beans and maybe a little water. At this point I would turn the heat right down or even off and make sure it was all mixed up. During the frying stage, there may have been some light burning or sticking of the onions or steak mince to the bottom of the pan. This can now be dissolved easily into the liquid by light scraping or just stirring, it will also add a lot of depth to the flavour!

For the next stage, put the lid on the pot and use it like a slow cooker. Place it in the oven on a medium heat or continue to cook on the gas on a very low heat, stirring occasionally and making sure there is not too much sticking to the bottom of the pot until it's done.

If you really wanted to save on the washing up, you could eat it right from the pot.... But this may be frowned upon. My mother would not be happy with me if she knew I was advocating this type of behaviour ☺

- **A metal sieve can be used for steaming veg separately at the same time as cooking**

If you are making a stew, paella or any one pot recipe that needs a side of steamed veg or steamed fish etc. You can easily create a steamer with your one pot. With a paella for instance, if you were going to be serving it with fresh runner beans or broccoli for example, you could put the veg into a sieve place the sieve over the pot and add the lid, this will create a steamer of sorts. Just remember to add a little extra water to your recipe to account for the gap that the sieve will create between the lid and the pot.

The sieve you use for this should be small enough to fit into your pot and fairly shallow. The best ones to use for this are also made of metal and should have a long handle and a rest opposite the handle so it can be placed in in suspension across the pot.

How much of a snack is this?

We've talked about meals and food type ratios, but what about snacks? There are pros and cons to snacking; it can be a good thing or a terrible thing.

There are two questions that you should ask yourself when deciding if your snacking is good or bad.

Is this a quality food?

&

How much of a snack is this?

If this is your first time venturing into the dieting for weight loss game, you may not even have considered the food that you eat here and there to cause any consequence. The odd biscuit with a coffee at work, the small handful of jelly beans from a "help yourself bowl" left on the side at your aunties house, the bag of potato chips thrown on to your order at the petrol station, the box of snacks to go with that movie.

Every time that you put food into your mouth, you are giving your body more fuel, and this adds up, the more you snack, the more energy you will need to use if you want to remain in a calorie deficit. One function of creating a food diary is to highlight snacking habits and this can be a very valuable exercise for many people, but we will cover this later in this in great detail.

The aim of this book is not to point blame at certain foods or habits or to advise severely restricted food consumption, one of the main goals is to spark food awareness and empower you, the reader with the knowledge to take control and make informed decisions with eating in general and snacking is a big part of the puzzle for a lot of people.

Eating little and often or snacking between meals doesn't have to be a bad thing, it can actually be beneficial, depending on your lifestyle and obviously, the nature of these snacks.

If you snack or graze on food a lot, and this is not the best food for your lifestyle, it can have a very dramatic effect on your weight loss goals and body composition. We already know that the higher quality the food is, the better it is for your body, but many foods that are considered snack foods, are convenient and also readily available are the opposite.

With this in mind, let's go back to the two questions that you should ask when choosing a snack food.

Is this a quality food?

You can determine whether the food that you are considering is a quality food by matching it to one of the "Food types" mentioned in the "four steps to weight loss success chapter" (Know the food section). You will probably find that most, all in some cases of the food that you think of as a snack fits nicely into the "Treats and cheats" type of food. Biscuits, chocolate, crisp, etc. if you are from the UK or cookies, chocolate and chips if you are from the US. ☺

This is hard to get bypass if you are not used to food prep, are not used to alternatives, or you have formed habits that rely on routinely eating these types of snacks. The easiest way to get around this is to cut out snacking altogether. This will undoubtable work for weight loss and it is certainly an option for some people.

While a clean break from low quality nutrition snacking is the right path for some people, it is not practical for others.

If you have a busy, active lifestyle, it may be more beneficial and convenient or even essential to snack throughout your day, so cutting out snacking altogether can have negative effects. If this describes you, it's important that you are snacking on the right foods.

It's tricky to identify and organise healthy snack options and also, as it is with eating for weight loss and body composition change in general, planning and prep is needed with snacking too. So make sure that you add your snacks to your shopping list!

If you are going to add snacks to your diet plan that fit with the quality types of foods, you can consider adding these to your shopping list:

- Beef jerky or biltong
- Mixed nuts
- Popcorn
- Rolled oats
- Mixed seeds
- Brown rice cakes
- Vegetable chips
- Natural peanut butter
- Cottage cheese
- Avocado
- Fresh fruit
- Humus
- Vegetables that can be eaten raw (carrots and celery are good options)

This list is an example of quality foods that fit the types mentioned earlier in the guide. It might be worth trying to match the food on the list with the type mentioned in the earlier chapter. Is it a protein, fat, complex carbohydrate or fibrous goodness?

There is a lot that you can do with this list in a prep sense, and it can give a lot of variety for the snacks you eat through the average day. As this is all quality nutrition, some of it is fairly dense. This means that although it will fuel you adequately and leave you feeling satisfied, if you eat too much of some of this, you can easily put on extra fat stores.

We now have quality snack choices, and this leads us onto the second question.

How much of a snack is this?

The very best way to get around this is to know how much energy is in the amount of food that you are eating as a snack. To get the most accurate estimate of what's right for you, you will need to go through the "level 2" section in this book "Advanced planning and macros". This will give you the tools needed to plan and prep the right portion size for all of your meals, including snacks for a full day. This sounds like a lot of upfront work, but if you are serious about getting actual results, it is well worth it, and it gets easier, the more you stick with it.

If you are not at level 2 yet or you are taking smaller steps on this journey, this is no problem. Here are a few good ways and things to consider when estimating whether you are eating the right amount that makes up a snack and not an extra meal:

- If it is fibrous goodness, you can eat more of this type of food than fats and proteins without over eating. So think carrot and celery sticks as fillers.
- If you are eating fats such as nuts and humus, a ½ cup is more than enough for a snack. The more that you use these measurements, the easier it will be to just estimate these portion sizes by sight.
- The same ½ cup measurement can be used for measuring out proteins such as jerky, biltong, or cottage cheese.
- If you are organised, you can invest in small, plastic pots that hold ½ cup measures and simply fill these every morning ready for the day ahead. This is another habit that is easier to get into than you may think.
- On certain food containers such as humus, cottage cheese, yoghurt or peanut butter, it may give a recommended serving size. For example, it might say "½ pot contains X amount of calories" or "This packet contains X amount of servings". In my experience, this is more

often than not a good indication of the amount of this food you should eat in one sitting and a good start if you are not looking to jumping into calculations just yet.
- Remember that you can add one food from every food type to each snack, but this will bump up the energy intake significantly.
- Remember that every snack is an energy intake, so make sure you don't "over snack". Mid-morning and mid-afternoon snacking is a good goal.
- My recommendation is try to stick to one food type when snacking, with a preference of protein. Protein will keep you full for longer, help maintain and repair lean muscle, and is more forgiving than fats if you get the portion size wrong. You can also add some fibrous goodness to your protein snacks if you need to.

To sum up:

The more you know about food and nutrition, the more creative you can be with snacks. There are limitless healthy, snack options available to us and I would always recommend that you look at some of these options.

To wrap up this section, here is a brief summary of things to remember:

- Look for foods that fit the food types: Protein, complex carbs, fats
- You can snack exclusively on a single food type or combinations.
- Take the time to learn portion size for each snack
- Two snacks per day is a good goal to have: (Mid-morning and mid-afternoon)
- Make sure your planned snacking food is on your shopping list and you have it ready for the week ahead.
- Prep and planning is often the make or break with snacking routine, as it is with meal planning in general. If you don't make sure it's available when you need it, you are putting yourself in a position where it's easy to make the wrong food choice.

Water & your body, an easy tweak for maximum return

Making a few minor changes to the way you take on fluid can be one of the easiest; most effective tweaks to your body transformation goals and is a classic example of a "quick win".

Your relationship with plain old fashioned water and how you fit this into your daily lifestyle is responsible for much in the outcome and progress of your weight loss plans.

The most important thing to understand about your hydration levels is that if you are properly hydrated, your body can function a whole lot better. The role of water in the body is to transport nutrients. So if we are following all the other advice about eating quality calories and nutrients, and we give our body a decent vehicle to transport this quality energy where it needs to go, all of our body's systems will work more efficiently.

This means that if we are correctly hydrated:

- We'll Be more alert and be able to concentrate better
- We'll have more energy
- We'll have better, more effective workouts
- We'll burn fat stores more efficiently
- We'll have clearer skin
- We'll be leaner.
- We'll detoxify a lot more efficiently

There are a lot more benefits to staying correctly hydrated, and there are obviously a lot of issues that can hamper your weight-loss diet progress if you are dehydrated and not taking on enough water. You just need to imagine the opposite of the benefits of hydration to get an idea of this.

With correct hydration levels, we won't really notice most of the benefits as they are happening in the background, but one of the most positive, significant physical side effects is the lack of water retention leading to actual weight loss.

If your body is used to running on little water, it will hold on to all that it can to maintain a balance. This means excess water weight and excess fat weight because if we are not hydrated correctly, our body is not functioning optimally.

If you are regularly drinking water and are hydrated all the time, your body will adapt and no longer need to store this excess water. There are two huge benefits from this one act of making sure you are always hydrated.

You will lose body weight as your body will no longer need to store water, and because your body will function more efficiently, a very welcome side effect will be an automatic increase in fat loss. Add the right amount of quality nutrition to this, a bit of regular exercise and consistency, and you have a recipe for exponential weight loss success.

As it is with the advice in all of my books, I have real life, personal experience to share, this time in the process of hydration levels in the human body working to drop water weight. I feel the need to preface this with a warning that this is NOT safe and is just used to reinforce and highlight how the human body reacts to hydration.

Competing bodybuilders when they are in show condition aim to be as lean and muscular as possible. This means dangerously low body fat percentages and even more alarmingly low hydration levels.

To non-competing bodybuilders, this sounds like madness. But as a former competing bodybuilder myself, I can tell you that this is state of mind and winning or getting into the best condition that you possibly can is the primary goal and nothing matters more, not even your health.

Most uninformed people who see a bodybuilder in show condition will believe them to be strong, powerful, fit and healthy when it's actually the total opposite. These guys on stage are at their weakest and most depleted. But to get this type of condition, there are a few tricks that you can play on the human body and technically manipulate the systems.

During the prep and hard training that a bodybuilder does in the lead up to a show, it's so important to stay correctly hydrated to make sure their body functions optimally while it is being fuelled with quality nutrition. But on show day, the bodybuilder only needs to look good, they don't need to function like they do on a training days.

One trick that a bodybuilder plays on the body to get that super lean look on show day uses water intake to manipulate the body to thinking it has too much water.

This is how it works: We know that the body likes balance. If there is too much water in the body, it won't store extra, there will be more frequent visits to the toilet and we will also look leaner, if the body isn't getting enough water, it will start to store it to maintain the balance.

This is what I did: After an extreme, twenty week fat loss diet of quality calories, hard training and optimal dehydration, my body and its systems were extremely efficient. Four days before the bodybuilding show, I started to "super hydrate". I drank about 10 litres of water in the first day and doubled it the second day. To reinforce the warning again, this is ridiculous, it is not safe and I would recommend no one to do this.

This "super hydration" tipped the water balance that my body is constantly aiming for, and so the "Too much water" action is taken. My body now had to cut off any function to store water and get rid of as much as possible to restore the balance.

As the body turns off the water storage system and pulls the plug on any water in the body, I then stop drinking altogether at the start of the 3rd day. My body was still working to get rid of the excess water and didn't know that it would not get any reserves. This is the manipulation of the body's system.

It was towards the end of this 3rd day that I saw a lot more definition appear in my legs in particular as the dehydration really kicked in.

The last part of this manipulation is to cause further dehydration. This is done by drinking half a bottle of white wine before bed and the other half first thing in the morning. I'm not sure there any other competitive sports where it's common practice to drink half a bottle of wine on the morning of competition day! Hopefully this goes further to highlight that this not a healthy or advisable process.

The diet and training that is aimed to strip away body fat and maintain muscle mass on the lead up to a bodybuilding show takes the longest time and relies on the body being hydrated. But once a bodybuilder has stripped away all the excess fat that they can, there is still an element of water retention that can take from the result and this is where a competing bodybuilder can find even more of an edge, after all, the body is made up of 70% water. There are even further measures that can and are taken by a lot of competition bodybuilders such as taking diuretics, but this is not something that I did and thankfully, this was more than enough for me to drop the water that I needed to.

My experience of this process was not a good one. I got headaches early in the 3rd day and had to take anti-inflammatory pills to get through this. I lost so much water that I didn't even sweat when I got too hot, and after the show I was absolutely exhausted, to where I nearly couldn't stand up.

On the day of the competition I was very lean and as show ready as I could have been. As soon as I started drinking water again, it took time for my body to balance out. As a result, lost most of my definition a few days after the show as my body switched back to "Storage mode". It was dehydrated, so it needed to store water. This balanced out again to find an equilibrium as I settled back into an optimum hydration routine within a few days.

Although this is not a good idea, is potentially very dangerous and most definitely not a healthy thing to do (I can't stress this enough), it highlights and proves that correct hydration has a key part to play in weight management and the body's ability and reaction to dehydration and hydration and this is worth knowing.

How do we know what an optimal hydration level is? Most people will be in the right zone if they aim to drink 2 litres of water per day and this is the amount that I always aim for. If drinking plain water is new to you, this might feel like a lot and it may take some time for your body to adapt. If this is the case, I would start with ½ litre or 1 litre in the first week and then add more each week until you reach the 2 litre mark. Maybe you end up drinking slightly over 2 litres, but from experience, I've found this to be pretty achievable for most people and it's a huge step in the right direction for anyone who doesn't normally drink water as part of their daily routine.

Other drinks

It would be a pretty bland world if our only fluid intake was water. Once you decide what your water quota is per day that should be the amount of plain water that you drink and should not be what you use to make coffee with, use it to boil rice with or turn it into anything other than pure water, with the exception of natural tea, with no milk or sugar.

To make this more appealing, or if you really do struggle, you could add a few slices of lemon, lime or both to give it a bit of life and to keep track of the amount, it's really smart and convenient to invest in or recycle a bottle that holds your planned daily amount and fill this every morning before you start your day.

We should consider all other drinks for energy content. For example, a cup of coffee with milk and sugar contains an amount of energy or calories. If you drink a lot of these, it adds up. Milkshakes, protein shakes, fizzy drinks, fruit juice, smoothies etc. should all be considered as food or energy intake.

To sum this up:

- Your body functions much more efficiently when it's optimally hydrated
- Stay hydrated to lose weight through water retention
- Make water intake a part of your daily routine. This action is one of the best things you can do for the least amount of effort for long-term weight loss
- Consider all other drinks for calorie or nutritional content

Exercise & diet for weight loss

We all know that diet and exercise are the magic ingredients for weight loss, but as it is with diet, so it is with exercise. There are so many exercise options out there to choose from and many claiming to be the best for you.

For the goal of fat loss and effective body composition change, there are only really two things to consider:

- The more you move, the more calories that you burn.
- The more lean muscle that you have on your body, the more calories you will burn.

With these two things in mind, it really broadens the horizons in terms of exercise options. If you are eating mindfully, eating the good stuff, you have a handle on portion control and you are keeping yourself optimally hydrated, by adding in a regular exercise routine, you are turning the results output dial up significantly.

What's the optimum training routine to achieve the Holy Grail in body composition change? Having more lean muscle than we have body fat is perfect for long-term weight management, as in this state our bodies are working with us to constantly burn energy.

If we have a strong cardio vascular system too, we will have better blood flow, bigger lung capacity and a slower resting heart rate.

Functioning and developing muscles and a strong cardio system make for a healthy body and mind. If you have never achieved this state before, it truly is life changing.

To get to this point, we need to work on our muscles with resistance and we need to also challenge our cardio vascular system. This means some form of resistance training and some form of cardio training.

Now we have narrowed it down to two forms of exercise, we can narrow it further to suit you, your lifestyle and your preference.

Cardio

Cardio can be anything that works your heart and lungs. Walking, jogging, cycling, dancing, skipping, cross trainer sessions. So pick something that you can do and plan to do this regularly. Cardio training that works to burn fat most efficiently are sessions of about 30 – 45 minutes sustained activity; this could be a steady state walk, interval training, or a cardio session that uses a variable intensity. The golden rule to effective cardio and fat burning is the amount of time your heart rate is elevated through exercise.

Resistance

Resistance can be any form of exercise that works against gravity and engages muscle groups. Think of lifting dumbbells, kettle bells, body weight exercises, Pilates, exercise band training. Again, pick something that you are most likely to enjoy and stick to. You should also make this a part of your routine and aim to train with resistance regularly.

An effective solution

The type of exercise sessions I consider to be most efficient for the goal of reducing body fat percentage and developing lean muscle is circuit training using compound exercises. This is quick, can use minimal equipment and is extremely efficient. This type of training method however might be a bit too advanced for some people, but there is always a way to progress to this stage and make this an exercise progression goal.

As this is a book based on diet, I won't go much further into this. But if you are looking for a training solution for your circumstance, I am more than happy to point you in the right direction. I've written several in-depth guides that cover several different training methods, including circuit training, home workouts with resistance bands, bodybuilding and running. There is something for everyone!

Please feel free to drop me an email if you need further advice, always happy to help.

Your very own companion guide

Before we get started on all the practical steps that section 2 has in store, it's worth a pause, in order to digest what we have covered so far. I also want to highlight a few things that are majorly important for success. Everyone has goals in health, diet and other areas, but too many people never realise these goals. I want YOU to be one of the success stories.

Since my transition to self-employment and self-publishing began back in late 2013, this journey has been one of taking on huge amounts of information and I can definitely relate this to my journey of dieting knowledge, body transformations, exercise progression and general health and wellness.

The coin can also be flipped and I can say that I have implemented a lot of my lessons from my journey in health, fitness and exercise to being self-employed and the process of self-publishing.

From all of this experience, I can attest to several facts that cannot be denied if you truly want success:

- You get out what you put in, this goes for brute force and will power as well as learning and adapting to personal challenges.
- You are responsible for your choices.
- Reading and learning information is a must. But if you don't act on what you learn, nothing will change.
- If you make a mistake, learn from it, move on and keep heading towards your goal.
- Invest in yourself. Take more time out to plan, learn and consider your path to your goals.
- Invest in resources if you need them.

Without accepting and making good on this list of facts, you will be very lucky to achieve what you set out to achieve.

If you are serious about hitting your goals and would like to take this a step further, I would like to bring up the companion book that goes with this guide again. By now you will hopefully appreciate the idea a bit more. The bottom line is that the companion planner will enable you to put a big tick against each of the above points.

This "workbook and journal" is a physical notebook to document your progress through the weeks of your journey and is a big empowerment boost.

If you would like a place to conveniently plan and record:

- Your weekly goals
- Your daily food and water intake
- Your meals and shopping lists
- New, healthy recipes
- Any mistakes you made and how you intend to overcome them
- Your overall weekly progress

Of course I would think you were even more awesome for buying another one of my products, but ultimately this is about you. The bottom line is that I want you to succeed and this companion guide is an excellent tool to use, refer back to and plan even further progression on your journey to success.

There is far more value to writing your goals and documenting your progress on a physical record than there is on a digital one, and this is my solution to making this process as easy as possible for you to follow

So if you would like empower yourself and grab your copy of:

"A diet book for weight loss success, The workbook & Journal,"

If you put an order in for your copy now, you have a few days before it gets delivered to re-read anything you weren't sure about that we have covered so far or maybe carry on with the book and get to grips with the more advanced planning.

A nod to body types & genetics

There is a body type theory or "scale" that was introduced sometime in the 1940s that's used in the health and fitness industry today. Knowing your body type according to this theory will help you understand the game a little better and possibly give you a slight edge.

Body types are essentially just another way of describing a "collection of genetics".

Genetics play a big part in how well we adapt to diet and exercise. We were all dealt a hand that we have to play with, but if you know the game, you can play your hand to maximum effect.

Before we get to section 2, I want to give a nod to body types and genetics. Although all the rules and the general approach of this book apply to everyone, regardless of body type, there are still certain things that you can know in relation to your body type that might enhance your results and make the food choices a more efficient fit for your ultimate goal.

With this said, I would like to make it clear that whatever body type you are, you can absolutely find a diet and lifestyle plan that aligns with your goals using the process in this book. The more that you know about yourself, the better equipped you will be to achieve your goals.

Everyone has a different genetic make-up, a different lifestyle, different set of ideas, likes, dislikes and so on. We do, however, all fit into a body type category.

We'll fit directly into, or be a combination of one of three body types and depending on where you are and what your goal is, you'll have some advantages and some disadvantages.

The three main body types are:

- Endomorph
- Ectomorph
- Mesomorph

We will look at these categories and match a well-known personality who is also great at what they do to each to help visualise.

I also want to precursor this part by saying that even though some body types are better at burning body fat and some are better at building muscle, each one of these body types can be out of shape and overweight if the diet and lifestyle is less than optimum. Each one of these body types can achieve amazing fitness results, even if their particular situation is at a disadvantage in relation to their fitness goal.

For fat loss, the same general rules apply to every body type but there are a few tricks that you can use to your advantage in the gym, or the kitchen that you can try in order to give you an extra edge and get to your goals more efficiently.

Ectomorph
The ectomorph is someone who naturally has a low body fat percentage, has long, slim limbs and has a hard time putting on muscle. With burning body fat, however, the ectomorph is better equipped to do so than the endomorph.

Some examples of pure ectomorphs are Ewen Bremner and keira knightley

Endomorph
The Endomorph will sometimes be referred to as "big boned". They are usually shorter and stocky and have a hard time losing body fat percentage. Endomorphs are however great at building mass and maintaining muscle.

Some examples of pure endomorphs are Melissa McCarthy and Jonah Hill

Mesomorph

The mesomorph is the middle guy. Naturally lower in body fat than the endomorph but thicker set than the ectomorph with a classic well-proportioned build. The mesomorph is good at putting on muscle and reasonable at burning fat. But will sometimes struggle to maintain muscle mass.

Some examples of mesomorphs are Michelangelo's David statue and Fatima Whitbread.

As mentioned, most of us won't fit directly into one of these categories, we will fit somewhere between them. Using myself as an example, I fit between the ectomorph and mesomorph categories. I have long limbs and if it wasn't for the long-term weight lifting and bodybuilding goals, I would have little muscle mass. My body type spills over to the mesomorph type however as I have a slightly bigger frame, but I don't burn body fat as well as a pure ectomorph.

For you, and where you fit, think about the traits of each body type and make your evaluation.

These are some questions to get started with:

- Are you tall (Ecto/ Mesomorphic trait)?
- Are you short or medium height (Endomorphic trait)?
- Do you have long, thin limbs (Ectomorphic trait)?
- Do you have short, stocky limbs (Endomorphic trait)? Do you have balanced proportioned limbs (Mesomorphic trait)?
- Have you always been on the overweight side (Endomorphic trait)?

Remember that you may fit between categories like me. So when you reach your decision, you can either take the eating habits of the body type that you feel you most likely fit into or you can use eating habits from both categories. This will depend on your goal, however.

Next, let's look at how we should eat as each of the body types.

Once you have determined where you fit on the body type scale, the next thing is to decide how to eat in relation to your fitness goal. For the purpose of this guide, we will focus on the goal of fat loss. I will also reiterate that this is an optional extra step that you can consider adding to your plan.

Whether you choose to follow this advice and actually implement it into your plan or not, it is definitely worth knowing where you fit and understanding your natural strengths and weaknesses. Having this knowledge and the awareness that it will give you is useful for making certain food choices in the future.

Here are a few tips and tricks that you can use with diet and training to give you an advantage based on the goal of fat loss for each body type.

Fat loss tricks for an endomorph

Food: Reduce portion size and calorie intake slightly more than the recommended. More food means more calories, and more calories have the potential to be stored as fat. This can be the biggest disadvantage for many endomorphs, as smaller portion sizes can often leave you feeling hungry.

Be more aware of calorie-dense foods types (fats in particular as these are easy to overeat) by changing the ratio of your food types to maybe cut fat to 10% and filling up on more fibrous goodness foods. Cutting any food ratios down can be tough for some, so have a play with the ratios keeping this in mind if you struggle here.

Food that fits the "Treats and Cheats" type also has a bigger negative effect for Endomorphs, so this is something to consider too.

Exercise: Focus on cardiovascular exercise every session or even every day. Walking at a fast pace or doing interval training will boost your fat burning efforts. Make sure that you are working at an intensity that causes you to get a light sweat on in these sessions to make them count.

Circuit training is a solid choice for resistance training for the endomorph. Focus on full body workouts when using circuits. Compound movements like squats, shoulder press, push ups and rows should be prioritised as each rep of a compound exercise works several large muscle groups at the same time and this intensity will help further with fat loss goals.

Fat loss tricks for an ectomorph

Food: Stick to the daily recommended calorie count and practice all the good stuff, but if you are a natural ectomorph, you will have a bigger margin for error when planning your diet. Natural ectomorphs will quickly see progress if they are doing the basics well.

Exercise: Weight training and resistance exercise, with a focus on strength and muscle building, should play a big part in an ectomorphs training plan. But cardiovascular exercise should not be totally neglected. Steady state cardio 3-5 times per week is a good starting point.

A well-designed exercise plan can have a big impact on body transformation goals for everyone, but for the Ectomorph, the impact is far greater when fat loss is the goal.

Fat loss tricks for a mesomorph

Food: Stick to the daily recommended calorie count and practice all the good stuff, but if you are a natural mesomorph, it's still important that you do the basics well and always keep a balanced and measured approach.

Exercise: A balanced mix of cardio and resistance training is a sensible approach. As a mesomorph, however, you can have a stronger focus on either cardio or resistance. Circuit training is always a good option for fat loss and muscle tone. I would suggest that if you prefer one training method over another, and this fits your goals, stick with it.

To sum the subject of body types up and reiterate the points I opened with, I want to again say that this part is just to give a nod to the fact that different body types and genetic make-ups can respond differently to diet and exercise, but the general rules, planning and all other parts of this book will work for everyone, regardless of their body type.

If you now see that your body type doesn't do you any favours when it comes to your fitness plans, this is not a problem. I can tell you that I have a lot of the ectomorph traits, and this did not play out well with my bodybuilding plans. Sure, I will never be Mr Olympia, but it also didn't stop me from competing as a bodybuilder and placing higher than people with better genetics than me.

Whoever you are, whatever your circumstance or genetic status, you always have the opportunity to be the best version of yourself.

SECTION 2 – Creating Your Diet

Introduction to section 2

Until now, we have just talked about the how's and the why's. This is great having all the information and it may be good enough for some people to go away and put it into practice, but I know if it were me getting into this I would need a lot more guidance. So in this section, we will go through the entire process of setting up your new diet plan.

By the end of this section, you will have a full plan that you can move forward with and get started on right away.

There's no doubt that diet, nutrition, new information, planning and prep can be very overwhelming when you start out. Jumping into a more advanced way of thinking right away is not helpful for most people who are beginning this journey, (me included) so section 2 will have two levels of planning and practical steps.

Level 1

Level 1 is designed for the total beginner. This will give you a solid plan that's easy to get started with and a generalised guide that utilises all the essential elements for weight loss success. If you have not had success with weight loss or had experience with diet planning before, you will find the advice and practical exercises more than enough to get started with. Starting off with the level 1 elements will also reduce your chance of overwhelm.

Level 2

Level 2 will give you everything that level 1 offers, but it will also give you a few extra tools to help you make the diet plan more specific to you as an individual with goal specific planning. It will also show you how to use more advanced ideas and use terms and techniques that many personal trainers will use when creating a diet for their clients.

Let's get right into the first step!

Step 1 - Start your food diary

Level 1 and 2

Creating a food diary is not only one of my first practical recommendations for people wanting a weight-loss diet, but it is also a recommendation that I would suggest for anyone who is interested in fitness and lifestyle changes of all kinds.

A food diary doesn't just give you a list of food that you've eaten in any given week. It can give you so much more insight into your habits, mistakes, types of food that you favour over others, water intake and give you ideas on small tweaks that can be made right away along with ideas for more substantial change.

In essence, this is a great exercise that helps you to identify where you are with your diet at the moment and then helps you make solid plans in order to achieve your goals.

As you can see, there are many benefits in doing this exercise and I've seen this to be an eye-opening experience for clients in the past. In this step, we will run through the process and I'll show you an example.

On the next page is a blank template that I've created. If you are reading the paperback version, you can simply write directly on the pages, and this is the same format that appears in the *"A diet book for weight loss success, The Workbook & Journal"* so it is familiar if you are following along and filling in your copy in real-time.

This is what the template looks like:

TIME	MONDAY	TUESDAY	WEDNESDAY	THURSDAY	FRIDAY	SATURDAY	SUNDAY
WATER							
05:00 - 06:59							
07:00 - 08:59							
09:00 - 10:59							
11:00 - 12:59							
13:00 - 14:59							
15:00 - 16:59							
17:00 - 18:59							
19:00 - 20:59							
21:00 - 22:59							

"How to" with the food diary

I am a big fan of having an old school pen and paper document as this can't be hidden away in a "cloud", tucked into a folder on a desktop to collect "cyber dust", or kept on an app that gives you the data only when you connect, this is a physical reminder of your goals and it's in your face for real accountability! So the reason for printing this out and writing on it is not because of my age or lack of technological knowledge, I know this to be effective!... If you are struggling to get a copy of one of these, I can fax one over to you ☺.

You will see there's a space to jot down everything that you eat and drink based on two-hour windows and for every day of the week. There is also a separate row for "Water".

I would suggest that you make at least two copies of this and fill it in for two consecutive weeks (Again, there are multiple copies of this in the companion guide "*A diet book for weight loss success, The Workbook & Journal*"). Make sure also that these weeks are "normal" weeks, meaning that it's not a holiday or Christmas as this will not be as useful. Most of us eat a lot more of the things that we wouldn't normally eat at times like Christmas and when we go away on a break.

Having two weeks of personal food intake to start with will give you a fair amount of insight into changes that we can make right away, and habits that we can work towards changing for habits that are more fitting to our goals.

It's best to start filling this in on a Monday, as you will have a full week of information on one page to look back at.

Once you have a physical copy of your "diet diary" ready to go, you need to decide on how much water you aim to drink. I always recommend that you have at least 2 litres per day. As we know, water plays a part in making us more efficient at everything, so this is important. Write down the amount you aim to drink each day below the day field on the sheet. Notice here that there is a blank check box here too. This is for ticking or crossing, depending on whether or not you hit your target. The rule here is that you either do or do not.

When you fill the chart in, write down everything that goes into your mouth that has calories or as we know it "energy". This includes, meals, snacks and drinks the only thing you can omit is plain water.

A common reaction is to sometimes "forget" to write on the sheet as it looks bad, but if you miss bits and pieces out, you won't be getting the most out of this and ultimately won't get your results. We are here to be honest with ourselves and see where we can fix problems.

Another tip here is when listing the foods you eat, list the individual foods that make up a meal, sandwich or snack and the amount. An example of this is that if you have a tuna sandwich, you would list the amount of bread (X amount of slices/ type of bread), the amount of tuna (X amount of grams), anything else that was on the sandwich such as mayo, salad, etc.

You can really do this with anything you eat, and it will be a lot easier to do this if you prepare your own meals rather than buy ready meals. More on this later.

So before you get started, here are a few bullet points to sum up how to go about this -

- Make sure you have at least 2 copies for 2 weeks' worth of tracking
- Start on a Monday
- Decide how much water you will drink every day (I advise 2 litres)
- Record EVERYTHING you eat or drink that has energy/ calories.
- List the individual foods that make up a meal/ sandwich or snack
- Be honest with yourself

Food diary example

Let's look at an example of how I would do this.

At the time of writing this book, I am thirty-eight years old and I'm not taking my training and diet too seriously. I am however training about 4 – 5 times per week on a bodybuilding routine in the gym to challenge all major muscle groups. I would not say that my diet is particularly strict and I would say that it is definitely not what you would expect from a performing athlete.

My approach is to make sure that I am not putting on too much excess fat while maintaining a fairly lean and proportioned physique through diet and exercise whilst also allowing myself regular, but limited access to the "treats and cheats" food types.

Over the years, I've learned how my body reacts to too many calories and not enough exercise and can identify when the balance slips. I know what to do to get back on track before it gets to a point where it becomes harder work than it needs to be. By understanding the foods you are eating and creating these diaries, you will be able to do this too.

So here is an example of a recent week for me, using the template

TIME	MONDAY	TUESDAY	WEDNESDAY	THURSDAY	FRIDAY	SATURDAY	SUNDAY
WATER	2 litres 😊	2 litres 😊	2 litres 😊	2 litres 😊	2 litres 😊	2 litres ❄	2 litres 😊
05:00 - 06:59							
07:00 - 08:59	½ cup oats, whey protein powder, ½ table spoon peanut butter	½ cup oats, whey protein powder, ½ table spoon peanut butter	½ cup oats, whey protein powder, ½ table spoon peanut butter	½ cup oats, whey protein powder, ½ table spoon peanut butter	½ cup oats, whey protein powder, ½ table spoon peanut butter	Bacon and egg sandwich (White bread + ketchup)	½ cup oats, whey protein powder, ½ table spoon peanut butter
09:00 - 10:59	Cup of coffee with sugar and milk	Cup of coffee with sugar and milk	Cup of coffee with sugar and milk	Cup of coffee with sugar and milk	Cup of coffee with sugar and milk	Coffee : sugar milk. Cheese on toast X2 + 4 cookies	Cup of coffee with sugar and milk
11:00 - 12:59	Protein shake	2 caramel rice cakes	Protein shake	Protein shake	Mackerel fillet, salad200g pretzel pieces	Chicken pasta, cheese	Protein shake
13:00 - 14:59	Tuna/ salad sandwich (2 slices Granary bread +mayo)	3 scrambled eggs, 2 granary toast	1 full egg/ 200ml egg white, 2 granary toast	Mackerel fillet, salad, 200g pretzel pieces	Cup of coffee with sugar and milk	Cup of coffee with sugar and milk	Cup of coffee with sugar and milk
15:00 - 16:59	Handful of peanuts	Handful of peanuts	Handful of peanuts	Meal out: Steak burger/ fries, coleslaw	2 cookies	Chinese takeaway, chocolate (Cheat night)	½ cup oats, cherry bio yoghurt,
17:00 - 18:59	Cup of coffee with sugar and milk	Cup of tea with sugar, soy milk	Chilli, ½ cup white rice				
19:00 - 20:59	Paella (Brown rice and salmon (butter), broccoli	Chicken breast, jacket potato (butter), broccoli	Cup of tea with sugar, soy milk	Cup of tea with sugar, soy milk, 2 cookies	Paella (Brown rice and salmon broccoli)	Cup of tea with sugar, soy milk	Chicken breast, jacket potato (butter), broccoli
21:00 - 22:59	Cup of tea with milk and 2 cookies	Cup of tea with milk and 2 cookies			Cup of tea with sugar, soy milk		Cup of tea with sugar, soy milk, 2 cookies

What's going on here?

Let's look at what's going on with this example

Water – I always try to drink 2 litres of water every day so I have filled this in on the "Water" row. Instead of giving myself a tick when I drank the target amount, it's a smiley face. After all, a smiley face can do a lot for your self-esteem! ☺. On this week I got 2 litres in on all days but Saturday.

Habits – When you have a weeks' worth of data in front of you like this, you will see some daily habits forming. The obvious one in my example is the first meal of the day. Every day is the same thing in the same time window. This is because it's quick, easy and full of the energy that I need for a normal working day and as I measure it with cups and scoops, I know how many calories and from which food types make this meal up. This is handy to know when or if you decide to take things a bit more seriously.

Breakfast habit -

TIME	MONDAY	TUESDAY	WEDNESDAY	THURSDAY	FRIDAY	SATURDAY	SUNDAY
WATER	2 litres ☺	2 litres ☺	2 litres ☺	2 litres ☺	2 litres ☺	2 litres ✸	2 litres ☺
05:00 - 06:59		½ cup oats, whey protein powder, ½ table spoon peanut butter					
07:00 - 08:59	½ cup oats, whey protein powder, ½ table spoon peanut butter	Cup of coffee with sugar and milk	½ cup oats, whey protein powder, ½ table spoon peanut butter	½ cup oats, whey protein powder, ½ table spoon peanut butter	½ cup oats, whey protein powder, ½ table spoon peanut butter	Bacon and egg sandwich (White bread + ketchup) Coffee : sugar	½ cup oats, whey protein powder, ½ table spoon peanut butter

There is also a "coffee habit" on there too, which we will talk about in the "possible quick wins" part. But this is still a habit and worth pointing out. You can see there are plenty of coffee's going in with sugar and milk and this all adds up to contribute to daily calories.

As you can see, it can be quiet a revelation to see your habits like this, and if you have over one weeks' worth of data, you will see habits forming on a weekly basis and then look to tweak things on a bigger scale. This would show for me on the weekends and especially on Saturdays!

Let's talk about Saturday – Saturday has been my "Cheat day" for years! This is the one day of the week where I eat what I want without giving it much thought. As you can see, there is takeaway food, chocolate and other treats and cheats in there. Personally, I find that this system works well for me as I can get stuck into my favourite treats and cheats while remaining guilt free. This does work for some people, but it can be a bit tough for others, so a "cheat day" is a personal preference.

Possible quick wins – Once you have completed a week's food diary, you will have something that looks similar to mine. This is a picture of your eating habits, the food you eat and the timings, etc. Now you can make a few changes with a better understanding of what it will look like in that picture. As mentioned before, you can make some long-term, substantial changes or you can plan for some "quick wins". The quick wins option should be the first thing that you plan to do.

"Quick wins" are small things that you might not notice as much but have a big, cumulative effect on your progress.

Using my food diary as an example to highlight this. If I wanted to lower my body fat further, there are a few things that I can do right away. In the picture of my food diary below, I have circled in red every time I had a coffee with milk and sugar. A quick win to my diet would be to ditch the sugar or that cup of coffee altogether. By losing the sugar and maybe finding an alternative zero calorie sweetener, I would cut out all of those extra empty calories.

TIME	MONDAY	TUESDAY	WEDNESDAY	THURSDAY	FRIDAY	SATURDAY	SUNDAY
WATER	2 litres	2 litres	2 litres	2 litres	2 litres	2 litres	2 litres
05:00 - 06:59							
07:00 - 08:59	½ cup oats, whey protein powder, ½ table spoon peanut butter	½ cup oats, whey protein powder, ½ table spoon peanut butter	½ cup oats, whey protein powder, ½ table spoon peanut butter	½ cup oats, whey protein powder, ½ table spoon peanut butter	½ cup oats, whey protein powder, ½ table spoon peanut butter	Bacon and egg sandwich (White bread + ketchup)	½ cup oats, whey protein powder, ½ table spoon peanut butter
09:00 - 10:59	Cup of coffee with sugar and milk	Cup of coffee with sugar and milk	Cup of coffee with sugar and milk	Cup of coffee with sugar and milk	Cup of coffee with sugar and milk	Coffee: sugar, milk. Cheese on toast X2 + 4 cookies	Cup of coffee with sugar and milk
11:00 - 12:59	Protein shake	2 caramel rice cakes	Protein shake		Mackerel fillet, salad 200g pretzel pieces	Protein shake	
13:00 - 14:59	Tuna/ salad sandwich (2 slices Granary bread +mayo)	3 scrambled eggs, 2 granary toast	1 full egg/ 200ml egg white, 2 granary toast	Mackerel fillet, salad, 200g pretzel pieces	Cup of coffee with sugar and milk	Chicken pasta, cheese	Cup of coffee with sugar and milk
15:00 - 16:59	Handful of peanuts	Handful of peanuts	Handful of peanuts		2 cookies		½ cup oats, cherry bio yoghurt.
17:00 - 18:59	Cup of coffee with sugar and milk	Cup of tea with sugar, soy milk	Chilli, ½ cup white rice	Meal out: Steak burger/ fries, coleslaw	Cup of tea with sugar, soy milk	Chinese takeaway, chocolate (Cheat night)	
19:00 - 20:59	Paella (Brown rice and salmon broccoli)	Chicken breast, jacket potato (butter), broccoli		Cup of tea with sugar, soy milk, 2 cookies	Paella (Brown rice and salmon broccoli)	Cup of tea with sugar, soy milk	Chicken breast, jacket potato (butter), broccoli
21:00 - 22:59	Cup of tea with milk and 2 cookies	Cup of tea with milk and 2 cookies					Cup of tea with sugar, soy milk, 2 cookies

You may have noticed that there are also smaller circles on the diary too. These could be another quick win as they are also empty, useless calories that I don't need. By making these two minor changes, I would be significantly helping the goal of fat loss.

More substantial tweaks – As well as minor changes, we can make big changes. The obvious one on my example is to ditch the cheat day altogether. This would make a big difference to my progress in in a positive way in a few short weeks if I had also made the suggested quick wins changes suggested.

More substantial changes can also build on what we already know. If you look at your example, you might see that there are a bunch of foods documented, but there are no values for these foods. There is no calorie count, and maybe there are no measures. If you find yourself in this position, it gives you a lot of potential for change. This is the time to start to measure out your food and understand the quantities you are eating.

You will notice that on my example, there is mention of "1/2 cup" and a "Handful of peanuts". This is because I know how much energy a ½ cup of certain foods give me and I have other things in place to measure out "a handful of peanuts". I have a small pot that I know holds 30g of peanuts and I simply fill this up.

I class this as a substantial change because it takes some work upfront and you have to find your systems, but once you do, it's a lot more accurate and will help you dial in on your goals.

Another example of a substantial change in my example would be a bit more of a lifestyle change. If I my goal was to increase muscle mass and bulk up rather than weight loss. I would need to eat more calories as a general rule. I could do this in a few ways; one, by increasing every meal size or the other way would be to add another meal every day, or both.

If I were to add another meal, it would make sense to eat earlier in the day, so my first meal would have to be between 05:00 and 06:59. This would mean that I'd have to make sure I got up earlier every morning, resulting in a bit of a lifestyle change.

So that's an example of how this works and a few ideas about what you can do with this information. It really is valuable stuff and as it is with everything, the more seriously that you approach this and the more commitment that you give it, the better the result. Your diet diary will look different to everyone else's and your habits will also be unique to you and your particular lifestyle, so this information needs to be adjusted to suit you and your specific goals.

Once you have a full week (or better, two weeks) of your food diary filled in and you want to make some changes, here are a few questions to consider to help you pinpoint actionable changes.

- Are there any foods I eat regularly that don't offer quality energy/calories?
- Do I have any quick wins that are obvious? Sugar in coffee, too many sweets?
- Can I create more of a routine?
- Can I cut down on the quantity of treats and cheats?
- Can I replace any bad habits with good ones?

The more positive changes that you can make, the better result you will get in a shorter time frame, but it is also important to understand that some changes can disrupt the lifestyle you have been used to. Changes may also take some adjustment to routine, and this is something that should not be overlooked.

Although it is entirely possible to pull your roots up completely and put them down in a totally different setting, my suggestion is always to treat this as a long term investment and make consistent small changes over time.

Your weight loss and fitness results may be slightly slower to achieve, but you will only have to concentrate on one or two changes at a time. This will have a huge, positive impact on the mental aspect of dieting, help you manage any lifestyle alterations more easily, and you will have the bonus of creating good habits along the way. These changes will have a cumulative effect and have a sound foundation to stand on.

Step 2 - Set your goals

While you are working on your food diary and collecting this data, you can move on to the next step. This is to make some clear, detailed goals.

Without the time spent on defining what you want to achieve and aiming for that result, you'll be limiting your chances of success substantially.

Think of throwing a ball to hit a target. If you can see the target, you have a good chance of hitting it. If you are in a pitch black room, can't see the target and throw the ball toward a best guess, there is a high chance that you won't get a hit. The odds are really in your favour if you can see what you want to hit.

You need to do three things in this step – Make a long term, week by week and a day by day goal.

A generic example of this that is:

Day by day goal:

Aim to eat no more than 2500 calories of quality, whole foods made up of 40% complex carbs, 40% protein and 20% fat and drink 2 litres of water per day.

Week by week goal:

Lose 4lbs of body weight every week with a focus on fat loss.

Ultimate goal:

Develop a set of 6 pack abs in the next twelve months

This exact example will fit perfectly into many people's weight loss goals and It's not unrealistic. If this fits with your goals, by all means, take it and use it as your own as it is.

Here is a breakdown of why this example is a good one and what you should look for if this doesn't fit with your own goals or would like something a bit more fitting to your personal set of circumstances.

Your goal should be specific

We briefly touched on this earlier, but now we can see it in action. It's better to define exactly what you want to achieve from a diet plan rather than having a general idea.

"I want to lose weight" is a goal, but with the example above, we can see how much we want to lose and where we want to lose it from. This shows in both long term and short-term goal.

With defining your goal, first you should decide what the very best outcome would be. Think about what you would want from a weight-loss diet or exercise plan if there were no limitations. This is how you create a long-term goal that's ambitious. A lack of an ambitious goal could be very restrictive to your potential.

Once you have defined your long-term goal, you can then identify your short-term goal; you should now think about the steps that you need to take to reach the long-term goal.

It's important to make these short-term goals realistic, so think about this carefully. As highlighted in the example, 4lbs of weight loss per week is very reasonable, but if you set your standards too high and decide you want to lose 10lbs per week, you will set yourself up for disappointment. So keep it realistic and think about what you can handle.

Ask yourself what you can realistically do to achieve this on a week by week and daily basis. Can you handle the short-term goals? Do you need to eat a certain amount of calories per day? Do you need to look at your food diary to make small, daily changes from this? Do you want to merge exercise and diet goals together?

You should have time frames or deadlines

Time scale is another really important part of planning. Having a time frame to hit your ultimate goal will help with long-term focus and adding further time frames to your short-term goals will help to stay focused on a weekly and daily basis.

If you have an ambitious goal that part of you thinks is impossible, you may be blind to the small achievements you earn that will ultimately be responsible for achieving your long-term goal.

This is why I recommend using a time frame to break things down. Lots of good days add up to good weeks and lots of good weeks add up to good months and years. If you can recognise your daily and weekly achievements, you will be winning or seeing success more frequently. This is huge for motivation and consistency.

Having a deadline can also be a powerful tool for motivation and focus, as this will give you a finish line to head towards. There is a true story from my past in the book "Marathon training & long distance running" that tells of a guy who could see the finish line become stronger and more driven than he had ever been but as soon as the finish line was taken away, he crumbled and gave up.

So when planning your short term and long-term goals, put a stake in the ground, aim to hit your goals by a certain date. If you can see the finish line, you will be stronger.

Re-set your goals

Goals and plans are always fluid, and it's good practice to understand this from the outset. Once you have your initial goals set up, you may have to tweak things as you go. This could be to change your daily, weekly or even ultimate goal, so be open-minded and flexible.

If you are having issues with implementing parts of your lifestyle to fit be able to hit your goal, you might have to make changes here so you can actually do what it takes to hit your goal.

An example of this: If your daily goal is to eat 2000 calories of quality protein carbs and fat, but you are used to eating 4000 calories of takeaway food every day and you really struggle to hit this daily goal in the first week because it's too much of a shock, you may want to change your daily goal calorie intake to 3000 calories as it's probably more achievable. Once you are used to this, you can then reset again to your original daily goal of 2000 calories of quality food. There are many "stepping stones" like this that you can use to get to a bigger goal or a goal that you are struggling with and this will be down to the individual, so be creative and if you get really stuck, drop me an email, Facebook message etc. and I'll be happy to give you some ideas.

You may also find that you hit a plateau with your progress. If this happens, you need to reassess and look at why. Your ultimate goal might change, you might hit your ultimate goal and feel lost. Is it time that you got another ultimate goal that's even more ambitious?

There are limitless situations where you might have to change your goals, but remember that having goals will give you focus and motivation. You will have an enormous advantage over others that don't set goals and are far more likely to see real weight loss success.

What are your goals?

Day by day goal:

....

Week by week goal:

....

Ultimate goal:

....

Step 3 - Plan your meals & water

Planning and prep of your meals does not just start each morning for the day ahead, there is much more to it than that.

You could have made the best diet plan in the world the evening before you start, and the morning that you jump into your plan and get ready to prep for the day ahead, you realise that your cupboards, fridge and pantry don't have the food you need to pull this off.

Before you actually eat the first meal of your new, long-term diet, you need to sit down and plan it out.

Step #1 Sort your water intake

As mentioned, this is one of the high value, low effort tweaks you can make to your diet that will give you multiple benefits. Therefore, it's the first thing you should implement in your planning. If you take nothing else away from this book, do this.

We established earlier that 2 litres of water is a good benchmark for most people. I would suggest that you make this your aim form the outset but this is your plan so if for whatever reason this does not work, work with what does. If you are not used to drinking water at all and two litres is a big ask, you can work up to this.

If you have read any of my other books or followed along with my exercise videos, you will know that I fill a two litre bottle of water which I aim to finish each day. You can do the same, you can recycle a bottle or buy a new water bottle made for filling and drinking, these are widely available.

Once you have decided on your target amount of water per day and you have a bottle to suite this, fill in the blank below:

I will drink .... of water every day

Step #2 Plan your daily meals

This is where you sit down with a cup of tea (or glass of water if you are still working on your 2 litre, daily quota ☺) and plan your meals for the week. It might sound like a big, daunting task but you can make it a bit easier if you keep it simple to start with.

If you're new to this, instead of trying to plan for seven different breakfasts, lunches and dinners along with fourteen different types of healthy snacks, you can plan for a single breakfast and have this every day, you can do the same for all other meals and snacks too. This will seriously lighten the load and get you into the routine with minimal work.

As the weeks go by, you can start to add different options in by trying new recipes and healthy cooking ideas that fit in with your diet plans. Before long, you will have a good variety of food that you are comfortable preparing and fitting into your life. You can even plan weeks of eating in advance, save them in a notebook and just decide to revisit them at the start of a new week.

Planning your meals is a big one so take the time to do this. The last thing that you want is find yourself hungry with no plans, no good food to hand and being tempted by the many convenient fast food options. This is not only a bad situation to be in from a diet point of view but it has a big knock on effect to the mental side of dieting.

Step #3 Make a shopping list

Working in synergy with your daily meal planning, a weekly shopping list prepared as part of your plan has plenty of benefits and is more helpful than it appears towards the success of your diet plans.

Once you have made your daily meal plan for the coming week, the shopping list creation and shopping itself is the easy part, you know what you need, so you just go and get it! This is an exciting part as it's the point where you commit to your next week of nutrition and you make it real.

Not only does a shopping list ensure you will have all the food that you need for the coming week, a shopping list will also help you avoid making bad choices when it comes to meal or snack times as you will have what you need when you need it.

Step 4 - Plan your exercise

Although it's possible to lose body fat percentage and change body composition by dieting only, I would always recommend that an exercise plan of some kind is used to compliment your nutrition intake and enhance the effect of the outcome.

As covered in an earlier chapter, we know that the more energy we use, the more fat we will potentially burn. If we have the right fuel, we will get the right result.

Everyone looking for general fitness and weight loss should find an exercise routine with some form of cardio and resistance exercise involved.

The exercise that you choose will however depend on your goals, so this is the first thing to think about. There are several steps to planning your exercise routine and you can do this by following the steps below.

Step #1 - Choose what type of exercise routine you want to follow and the intensity.

Think carefully about the outcome you are looking to achieve. If you would like to work towards a lean, toned and balanced physique, look into a balance of resistance and cardio using compound movements as the example in the chapter "Exercise & Diet For Weight Loss" highlights. This approach to training is an excellent choice if you've never had an exercise plan before. Training in this way is probably the best foundation for every other type of exercise goal.

If, however, you have exercise goals that are more specific, tailor your training to align with this outcome.

It's also important to make sure that you get the right training intensity for your fitness levels. You do not want to pick a training method or routine that will put too much strain on your body or is too much more advanced that your current physical ability. It's ok to have ambitious goals, but this is where training progression comes in. We all start somewhere.

On the flip side of this coin, if you are physically active, strong and cardio fit but you are looking to lose a bit of body fat for instance, you want to pick an exercise routine that will challenge you.

Either way, remember to decide on exercise that aligns with your goals. If you want to be a runner, chose something more cardio based, if you want to be a bodybuilder, choose something more resistance based, but it's always advised to have some form of cardio and some form of resistance exercise with any routine, even if you and your goals favour one over the other.

So take some time to think about what you would like to achieve from an exercise plan and fill in the blank:

The exercise routine, training method or programme that I will choose is:

....

Step #2 - Choose frequency of your exercise

Next up is to decide how often you are going to exercise. Obviously, the more frequently you can exercise the better, within reason. Moderate intensity training three to four times per week is recommended if you want to make a significant difference to your body composition.

Training every day is possible, but I would suggest that you have at least one rest day. Training is important, but when training consistently, it's also important to factor in rest days because your body needs time to repair and recover. With this "R & R", your body can use the quality nutrition that you are giving it to get ready to tackle the next training session.

If you plan to train three to four times per week, try to space these sessions out. A pattern such as Monday, Wednesday and Friday as your training days is optimal for the beginner or all over body workouts.

Although this is not practical for many people, some exercise is better than none, so training sessions should slot into your life where they most conveniently fit.

You may be following a specific routine or progressive training program that you have to make lifestyle adjustments for, such as getting up an hour earlier in the morning on training days, or going to bed later. If you are going down this route, this is outstanding! It's these types of commitments that really make the difference.

So, once you have found a training routine or method that you would like to follow, you can fill in the blank below:

The amount of times I will exercise every week is:

....

Step #3 - Choose the time of your exercise

Planning the time of your exercise sessions is a two-part thing; the time of day you plan to exercise at and the time you plan to spend exercise for. As you can see, to fill this in you must have filled in the other two steps.

Depending on your lifestyle, the exercise routine that you plan to follow, your level of commitment to exercise and where you have decided to fit your training in, there is a certain amount of dictation to this.

Most pre designed exercise routines will be around 30 minutes to an hour long, so if you are following one of these, this is the time that you will exercise for. If you are not and you plan to do your own thing, I would suggest that the time of your exercise should be in this frame with a minimum of 30 minutes and maximum time of an hour.

The time of day is totally down to you and your circumstance. I would advise that you fit this training in where it is most convenient to you. Training immediately after your working day, at lunch time or just before you start work is a solid plan as it fits with your current routine and works as a kind of extension to your normal, whereas if you decide to fit your exercise in to another part of your life, there will be more friction in making this habit stick. We are looking for long-term, consistent actions with diet and exercise. This is where the magic happens.

Once you have decided how long your training sessions will be and how long they will last for, fill in the blank below:

I will exercise on .... every week and these sessions will last.......

Level 2 (Advanced planning and macros)

This book is a guide for beginners, but I feel that I would be remiss if I did not explain how you can take things to the next level. In this section we will look at how you can go all in and act with the calculation of an old school, professional personal trainer who wants to get the very best for their client. Of course, you can also be the client!

If you follow this section, you will have the most accurate start to a new diet when it comes to the macronutrients and calories from the food you eat. You will also learn a lot more about the process and theories of calories in vs calories out along the way.

The first advancement from level 1 to level 2 is a change in thinking for the "types" of food. If you were paying a personal trainer to prepare you a diet plan with weight loss in mind, and you were to trust in their advice, you would probably expect there to be a plausible explanation available to you from them if you asked for it. So from here on in, we will use "industry standard" terms. The first term we will use is Macro nutrients or "macros".

Level 1 had us categorising foods into one of the five types based on that foods most abundant property. Salmon for example would be placed in the "protein type", nuts would be placed in the "fat type" and potato would be placed in the "complex carbohydrates type".

This is a great start and when practicing portion control alongside this method, it can work really well, and to be fair, it's all that many people will need to earn the results they are after, but we can be a lot more accurate if we want to step it up a gear.

Let's take a portion of salmon, for instance. We know that salmon is a source of protein, but it is also a source of fat. We know that fat has a significantly larger amount of energy (calories) per gram than protein and complex carbohydrates. This is where you need to start for taking it to the next level.

Breaking down each food further into the types it comprises is the next step. While we are here, and we are getting more scientific, we can address the "types" as "macros" (macro nutrients) instead. We will still focus on protein, carbohydrates and fats as these macros, but by breaking down each food into the macros they are made up of will go a long way in making things more accurate.

When we look at the macros in a 115g portion of salmon (this is a sensible portion size for 1 person in one meal), we see a breakdown of macros that looks like this:

115g of cooked salmon fillet:

- 28g protein
- 7g fat
- 0g complex carbohydrates

With this information, and because we know that there are 4 calories per gram of protein and 9 calories per gram of fat, we know that a 115g portion of salmon also gives us 175 calories.

28 (g protein) X 4 = 112 calories from protein

7 (g fat) X 9 = 63 calories from fat

112 (calories from protein) + 63 (calories from fat) = 175

Looking at food with this much detail will give us a much clearer idea as to the amount of energy (calories) that we are putting into our bodies.

In advanced planning and macros, there are four pieces to the puzzle:

- BMR
- Calories
- Macros
- Diet plan based on macros needed

Step 1 - Work out your BMR

BMR stands for "Basal metabolic rate" this is a term that estimates how many calories a body needs to maintain and function at rest. This is kind of the industry standard for putting together a diet plan. Finding out how many calories you burn on a daily basis is a very valuable piece of information, because if you know how much fuel your body needs, you will have a better idea of where to start with fat loss, muscle gain and any other sports specific fitness goals.

Although it's an estimate, it's probably the most accurate start that we can get with the tools we have.

BMR is calculated using your gender, weight, height and age. I have seen several ways to calculate BMR using different figures. Each method of calculation produces a result that's within a few hundred calories of each other. There are plenty of BMR calculators online that you can just put your stats into these days and it will do the working out for you. By all means, use one of these calculators as it will give you a starting point.

You can even calculate your BMR through all of the methods you can find and take an average. Having an estimated figure to start with is the main goal here.

For the purpose of this book I will use the method of calculation that I learned and have used with my clients in the past:

- Measure your height in centimetres and times this by 6.25
- Measure yourself in Kilograms times this by 9.99
- Add the two results together (Make a note of this number)
- Times (X) your age by 4.92 and take this number from the result you got from the previous step.
- Add (+) 5 for males or minus (-) 161 for females.

The formula will look like this:

If you are Male:

(MALE) BMR =

(Height in CM X6.25) + (Weight in KG X9.99) – (Age X4.92) + 5

If you are female:

(FEMALE) BMR

(Height in CM X6.25) + (Weight in KG X9.99) – (Age X4.92) – 161

This gives us an estimate of the amount of calories our body needs if we stay at rest in a single day. Of course there are some methods that can give a more accurate figure, but this will require specialist equipment and laboratory conditions which are not available to most of us.

Step 2 – Harris Benedict equation

Once you have your estimated BMR, you need to link this into your lifestyle. If we are both the same age, gender, height and weight, we would get the same result for BMR, but I might work at a desk all day and have no interest in exercising and you may have a manual job and take part in regular exercises classes.

From this basic example, you can see that you would use a lot more energy every day than I would be, so you should take on more fuel to function.

This is where the good old "Harris Benedict equation" comes in, and it's the next calculation that takes our BMR and activity level into account when determining the amount of energy we need to maintain our current body weight.

Here are the equations -

If you do:

- little to no exercise, your daily calories needed = **BMR x 1.2**
- Light exercise (1–3 days per week) your daily calories needed = **BMR x 1.375**
- Moderate exercise (3–5 days per week) your daily calories needed = **BMR x 1.55**
- Heavy exercise (6–7 days per week) your daily calories needed = **BMR x 1.725**
- Very heavy exercise (twice per day, heavy workouts) your daily calories needed = **BMR x 1.9**

This guide will give you an estimated figure showing how many calories that you should eat to maintain your current body weight.

Once you have an estimated figure, you have the power to test, change and own your diet.

Using me as an example

For the sake of clarity, I will show this formula working on myself with my current stats. For some perspective, I am average height but slightly above average build at the time of writing as I train to maintain muscle mass with bodybuilding style workouts.

Step 1 – My BMR:

- Male
- Height = 178cm
- Weight = 89kg

So my calculation for step 1 looks like this:

$$(178 \times 6.25) + (89\ KG \times 9.99) - (Age\ 38 \times 4.92) + 5$$

BMR = 1819.65

The estimated amount of calories needed for my body to maintain and function at rest is 1819.5 calories per day.

Step 2 – Harris Benedict

Moderate exercise (3–5 days per week) Daily calories needed = BMR x 1.55

So my calculation for step 2 looks like this:

$$(BMR)\ 1819.5 \times (Harris\text{-}Benedict)\ 1.55$$

HB equation = 2820

The estimated amount of calories needed for my body to run and maintain based on my activity level is 2820 calories.

This figure gives me a great starting point. It tells me I can eat 2820 calories every day to maintain my current weight.

Whatever figure you end up with, it is worth mentioning again at this point that the recommended daily calorie intake for the average male is 2500 and 2000 for the average woman. If you are eating well over this and would like to drop body fat percentage, this is a solid starting point.

How to use this figure

I feel that the point of this being "an estimate" should be further reinforced here because there are a few factors that can have a sway on the accuracy of the estimate from person to person.

The obvious variable that may cause concern with this method is that the equation doesn't consider the individual's body composition. Maybe you are made up of 15% body fat while I'm 35% body fat, but we could weigh the same, be the same height and age. This would put our BMR at the same figure.

If this was the case, the calculation would under estimate calories for you and it would over estimate calories for me. To be clearer, this is less accurate for people that have very high body fat percentage and likewise for people who are on the leaner side.

With that said, this is still a great foundation and starting point for everyone. It's just worth pointing out to highlight the fact that the equation is still an estimate and that a bit of trial and error should be factored in as it should with any diet method.

With this in mind, here is an approach that you can take once you have your figure.

- Look back at your food diary and work out how many calories you are eating on a daily basis if you can.
- Get your calories from whole, quality foods
- Plan your daily food intake to be 200 calories below this figure, monitor for a week and then reduce in 200 calorie increments until you are losing around 4lbs per week

- Revisit the calculation when your weight changes.

Step – 3 Where do you get your calories?

Once you know what your BMR is and you have your estimation for daily calories needed to maintain according to the Harris Benedict equation, you can then break it down a bit further. You can work out how many calories of each of the three macros we have been working with that you should be eating daily.

We know that whole, unprocessed, quality food is the best for us so I will assume that this is a given, but we also want to work out the percentage of calories in our diet to match the recommended ratios that we covered earlier in the guide.

Calories from complex carbs – 40%

Calories from proteins – 40%

Calories from fats – 20%

So using me as an example again, I would take my estimated maintenance calorie intake of **2820** and do the following sums to quickly work out the percentage of daily macros:

2820 X 0.40 = 1128 calories from Protein

2820 X 0.40 = 1128 calories from carbohydrates

2820 X 0.20 = 564 calories from fat

When working out your calculation here, use either your maintenance figure or the figure you ended up with after any reductions. For example, if you decided to take 200 calories from your total to start with, use that figure.

If you follow the steps above, you will get an excellent idea of how your body reacts to the diet you have chosen. The information that you get from this will also give you a great starting point for any goal that you wish to pursue, whether this is fat loss, muscle building, maintenance, etc.

Here is the quick breakdown of how you should approach this process:

- Stick to eating your estimated amount of calories
- Are you losing body fat after 2 weeks?
- Yes – Winning! Keep going until something changes. When it does, carry on the process.
- No – Re assess your food choices
- No – add more exercise OR take away 200 calories from your current, daily quota.
- Making sure these calories come from quality, whole foods. Test this for at least two weeks and monitor results. If you are not losing body fat, revisit your calculation.
- Keep in mind the variables that count – Quality calories in: Good food and food volume. And energy output: Exercise intensity and frequency. These variables can be changed individually or simultaneously.

I would suggest if you fall into the very overweight category, that you use your BMR only without adding the Harris-Benedict equation as your start point.

I will point out again that this is just an estimate, a base line for you to start with. You may find that you get it spot on first time, if that happens, great!

However you may find that after several weeks of the changes being made, you have not lost or gained; it is then time to add or subtract another 10%, the longer you perceiver with this, the more valuable that the information will be to you.

TO SUM UP THE FORMULA

To Sum up what we have just covered, I have listed the steps that you need to follow in order to plan your diet:

- Weigh yourself and measure your height.
- Work out your BMR.
- Add the Harris Benedict equation.
- Make adjustments to this figure if you feel it is an over estimation (take 200 calories each week)
- Work out where your calories come from. Aim to eat whole, nutritious, quality foods.
- Split calories into meal sizes according to the amount of times that you plan to eat per day.
- Stay consistent with this for around four weeks, then reassess and make changes.

Keep going! Optimise for success.

Once you have your plans in place and you start going, you will undoubtable come up against setbacks. This is normal. Maybe there are parts of your plan that don't fit in to your lifestyle; you may find there is an issue with the prep of the meals you planned to eat. A lot of unforeseen problems can pop up, and therefore we need to be fluid and adaptable with our planning.

There is also an outcome that will have us changing our plan because we have out grown it and progressed. If we hit a plateau, it's time to revisit our goals, look at how we can tweak our diet and exercise routine for further progress and new challenges.

Diet, exercise, healthy habits and routines are all work in progress. We can always improve on our situation and it's up to us as individuals to decide where we want to be and make changes that will steer us towards our goals.

Always remember why you started, look for and identify your problem areas and do what you can to reduce or remove them. Consistent, sustained small changes that are extremely powerful, so if you make a small, positive change that you think is insignificant at the time, think again, this is huge!

Thank you and goodnight!

This is the first book that I've written on diet, but it's been a project that I've wanted to get stuck into for some time. The reason for holding off was because of the hugely contradictory nature of diet for weight loss. Add the subjective nature of the topic to this, and it makes it hard to write a guide to suit everyone.

There are many diet theories that will give the same results, but I wanted to write a guide that focuses on the "basics done well". Everything in this diet book will apply to most, if not all. I hope that this has given you a base to work from, shown you that basic knowledge, a willingness to learn and a little upfront work can lead to truly amazing results.

Above all, I hope this has left you with a feeling of empowerment and positivity that will set you up for exponential success with weight loss.

If you are looking for an exercise plan that suits your needs and aligns with your goals, I have also written several exercise guides in specific niches, again, all based on personal experience. So please go and check these out if you are in the market for a new training routine.

I would like to wrap this guide up by thanking you for your purchase; The sales of my fitness books are at the time of writing, my sole income, so you made my day when you clicked the "Buy now" button! You are the best!

Sales and Amazon reviews mean the world to me so if you want to help me out even more, you can go back to Amazon and leave a short review and a star rating. I always feel bad about asking for reviews but I'm a self-published author and to get anywhere in this game, you need reviews, so it's a necessary evil.

I appreciate the time that you have invested in my work and I will do all that I can to help you out more. If you have any questions or would like to bounce some ideas off me, please drop me an email –

Jim@JimsHealthAndMuscle.com I want to see you succeed with your fitness and weight loss plans and it's always great to hear from readers like yourself.

Motivation is the driving force!

If you enjoyed this guide, you like the style and want more in the way of fitness; I have already published a fair few books on the subject. There is something for everyone!

I would like to leave you with the opening chapter from one of my favourite – "Fitness & Exercise motivation".

This was a joy to write, and I've made many new friends as a result of publishing this book. It's been great to connect with readers (and listeners of the audio version) too!

Motivation is the driving force behind any fitness result but it is precious! If we lose it, we lose our way! This book was written not only to help maintain the motivation, but to turn it into an unstoppable force that guarantees our success!

Here's the opening chapter...

"Fitness & Exercise Motivation": By James Atkinson – excerpt

It's a cold dark day in October, the rain is lashing down with no signs of stopping; the wind is howling and the hope of a peaceful, warm summer's morning seems like worlds away.

From a warm cosy flat whilst sipping on a hot coffee, he stares out of the window at the torrential downpour and the stoic leafless trees that are being brutally assaulted by the relentless wind. He weighs up his options. He could sit back down, get another coffee on, and maybe even make something nice to eat. It is Sunday morning, after all.

Or he could do what he had planned to do, get out there and make the journey to the gym on his bike to complete his last training session of the week. After some hesitation, he recognises he has come too far to take the easy option and give it a miss. With a reluctance bought on by the thought of what he is about to endure, he puts on his training clothes, fills a bottle of water and heads down the stairs to his waiting transport.

The bike leans up against the shoe rack. It is an old and well-used thing that was given to him by a good friend a year or two ago. There are plenty of scuff marks on the frame and a fair few rust spots, but it has never let him down. At least this vital piece of kit would not be a target for thieves. With this in mind, he is aware of a smile on his face. He quickly puts on his waterproof coat, throws on his backpack, and opens the front door.

He wheels the bike out into the pouring rain and while holding the seat to steady the bike with one hand; he closes the door with his free hand.

"I'll see you soon" he mumbles to himself as he pulls the elastic draw strings of his hood a bit tighter around his neck. A few minutes later he is on his way to complete his training session. There is no turning back now, the hard part is over!

To some people, this little story may seem extreme and most would not need to ride a bike to the gym in the pouring rain to get their workout done, but the messages in this anecdote are at the heart of any fitness success story. If you can be the trainer or dieter that is serious enough about their goal to get out there and act with no excuses, you will be rewarded.

The easier it is for you to overcome stepping out of a comfortable environment into the pouring rain, choosing brown rice instead of white pasta or even starting your home workout routine, the easier it will be to reach, surpass, and maintain your fitness goals.

In this book, I will show you how.

Hi, I'm Jim, and yes, I am the guy who bikes to the gym in the rain and I have achieved a fair amount when it comes to developing my own fitness. But I would not say that I have a special gift or a secret that I used to give me an advantage over anyone else that would like to do the same.

Since my early teens I have been involved in some form of fitness training which has taken me from long distance running, bodybuilding competition, and I also served a number of years in the British army in an airborne unit (9 para sqn R.E).

As most people know, long distance running and bodybuilding competition are polar opposites when it comes to training routines and body condition, and I am not genetically built for either. So why is it that I can go further than most when it comes to reaching fitness potential? I believe that anyone can achieve great things in the fitness and fat loss game, there are no magic bullets, ultimate training routines or secret formulas to fitness and fat loss success.

The key is to become responsible enough to get yourself to where you are more than self-motivated enough to make the decision to step out into the cold and rain and make it happen!

In this book I will share my personal experience with some lessons learned that have been invaluable to me, along with some practical advice when it comes to overcoming the mental challenge that is at the crux of any fitness success story.

I base this advice on my personal experience of over twenty years in the health and fitness arena.

"Fitness & Exercise Motivation": By James Atkinson – Excerpt ends

JAMES ATKINSON

FITNESS & EXERCISE
Motivation

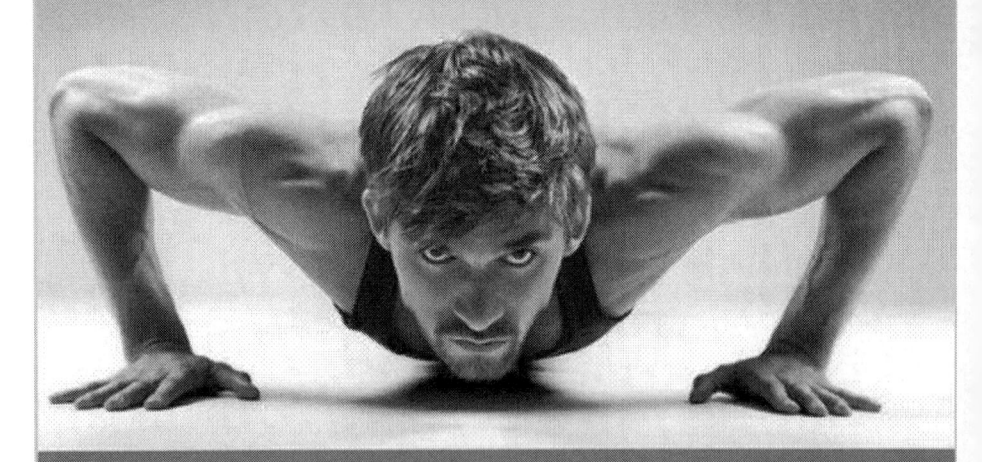

FITNESS SUCCESS TIPS FOR MIND-SET DEVELOPMENT AND BESPOKE FITNESS PLANNER CREATION

Printed in Great Britain
by Amazon